HOW TO

FEMINIZE YOUR FACE

Makeup and Hair Styling

(a helpful guide)

By

Martine Song

First Published in 2020

ISBN 9798552053032

Disclaimer

The following text contains various suggestions for feminizing your face using makeup and hairstyling techniques. Various products and techniques can irritate the skin, always check the labels and be aware of any possible allergies you may have. The author is not a trained counsellor or therapist for transgender issues or medically qualified. If you are seeking permanent transition or hormone treatments or surgery of any kind, please consult with a qualified practitioner. The author accepts no responsibility or liability whatsoever for your feminization activities.

Contents

Part I
The Female Face

"A woman should have many faces through her life, not just one face, not just one hairdo, not just one way. You want to keep rediscovering what's fun for you. "

Sharon Stone.

"In order to be irreplaceable, one must always be different."

Coco Chanel

Chapter 1 Introduction

Hi and Welcome. The theme for this volume is male to female transformation. Specifically, how to use makeup and hair styling to feminize your face. In the following pages all the differences between male and female faces and how to overcome them are explained. We will also consider the use of hair and accessories like ribbons, clips, and jewellery to pretty-up your look and bring out your femme personality. In other words, give your femme persona that little extra something that defines someone as not just female but also feminine.

Every woman has a certain elan. A style, energy, and enthusiasm for life that feeds into her look and personality. The sum is greater than the parts. If you have ever been beguiled by the laugh or smile of a woman, the language of her eyes, the way her hair falls across her face, or how she tucks it behind her ear, you will know that putting on your face is *so much more* than just slapping on some lippy, eyeshadow, and a wig. A successful and convincing male-to-female makeover relies on mastering the four pillars of feminization: face and hair, body and movement, fashion or style, and voice. This volume covers the first of these foundations and dips into ideas of fashion and style. The remaining pillars are discussed in sister volumes to this one.

A starting assumption is that you are completely new to feminization. We start right back at the beginning and develop all those little techniques that females learn from their moms, aunts, sisters, girlfriends or by experimentation to develop from gauche girls into confident classy women. There are many differences between the underlying structures of the male and female face. If you ignore them, no matter how much time you spend on your makeup, you will still be a kind of Aunt Sally or refugee from a Punch and Judy show. *We don't want that, do we?*

If you are already an established dresser or in transition, stripping back your technique to the basics is a good way to identify and overcome difficulties or refresh a tired look. Read these pages with a new eye and you will find some additional tricks, tips, and further insights to perfect your own method. Likewise, If you are a sympathetic female, partner, or a mistress interested in feminizing your man, you will be able to complement what you know already by taking into account the differences between the male and female face. Indeed, why not just give your beau this book as part of their training so they can learn for themselves.

Your inner girl

Carl Jung, the famous psychoanalyst, coined the terms Anima and Animus to describe the unconscious female and male parts of a person. He believed in a universal unconscious that we could all tap into that contains the feminine (and male) qualities we see in people. The Anima contains all the unconscious feminine psychological qualities that a man possesses. And, likewise, the Animus is a woman's unconscious male qualities. Jung thought that males were more likely to repress these qualities and that they were prone to come out in dreams and desires or influence how a man would react to the opposite sex.

If you haven't made contact with your female part yet here is a short mindfulness exercise. Try it if you like. You might be surprised at the outcome. Find a quiet spot, assume a comfortable position, close your eyes and regulate your breath so it is nice and even and not too fast. Let your body relax and your mind settle. When you feel comfortable visualize a small hut in a safe place (maybe a clearing in the woods or on a hill or a little fairy tale place). As you approach the hut invite your Anima to appear. Ask her to come out and talk with you. She might be a little coy or shy and need encouragement. All those years of hiding her away have made her extra cautious. When she does appear, take a moment. Look at how she dresses, what her hair is like, and how she moves. That is your inner girl and how she wants to be. You might find it all a little emotional. Give her a hug.

If all that sounds a little woo-woo and not for you that is fine. If you are drawn to feminization your Anima will exert her influence in other ways. You may not feel completely happy in yourself until you let her come out and play. Women have developed lots of tricks and techniques to dress for their moods and make themselves look more appealing, sexy, sensual, sophisticated, or cute. We will show you how to do all that so you can get the look you want and satisfy your inner girl.

Why feminize your face?

So, now is a good time to ask why you want to get into all this makeup and hair stuff? Well, duh, because you want to look like a girl, right! Well, not really. Most people just want to be happy. There can be a whole bunch of reasons why being more femme will create that inner happiness from naughty fun through to a 24/7 lifestyle. Here are a few that may resonate with you:

24/7 girls: in this first case you are dressing all the time and taking hormones with a view to transitioning permanently as female. Makeup and hairstyling will be a natural part of your lifestyle. We use the phrase Tgirl to differentiate those that have some surgery (aka a boob job) but stop short of the full transition through gender reassignment. You may know them more colourfully as Lady boys or Chicks with Dicks. The objective here is to be as authentic as possible so you will want to make your face up and style your hair like a regular girl. Without surgery you may find that you need to work to hide some of your male features. We will look at all the differences between male and female faces in later chapters so you can get the best look you can.

Drag Queen (or performance artiste). In this case you are not necessarily trying to hide your masculinity but celebrate the fusion of the male and female together. Here the makeup colours tend to be more garish and strident both softening and bringing out some of your male features. Stage performers can look devastatingly attractive, but they need the strength in colours to reach out to the audience. Especially in venues like night clubs where the lighting is subdued. Likewise, if you are a trans model or enter a Tgirl beauty pageant you will need to think about slightly darker foundations and crisper lipstick than usual to avoid your pretty features washing out under the bright stage lights. Modern makeup has its roots in the grease paint of the theatre but both these looks can be a little much when you are out and about in the shopping mall.

<u>Crossdressers:</u> we use this term as a catch-all for people that dress occasionally be it for social reasons or for naughty fun. In the former your goals can be similar to 24/7 girls though normally you won't have had any surgery or be taking hormones. You might want to glam up to go clubbing, enjoy some time shopping, or other outings. So, an objective is to be passable. That is, without any obvious 'tells' that you are male underneath. Alternatively, you may just want to potter about in your own home, cook, do housework, or hobbies so a simple look will be sufficient. The feel of girly hair and makeup will add to your femme feelings but how far you go with the techniques will be up to you. If your objective is just some naughty fun, the main reason to femme up is because you get aroused. It might be something you only ever do in the bedroom. Maybe just wearing stockings and lingerie are your thing. A hair piece and some rudimentary makeup skills could be all you want or need. You might like to develop a cheeky pinup girl, playboy model or 'Victoria Secrets' look.

<u>Gender bending</u>: in this case you might identify with being non-binary or even a bit of each. You want your face to represent that androgynous look between male and female. Or maybe you just want to break conventions and create an edgy different look with glossy lipstick or wear your hair in a girl style. Think here of Boy George in the Culture Club days, Adam Ant -if you remember him or modern-day comedians like Eddie Izzard (who referred to himself as somewhat boy-ish and somewhat girl-ish) or crossdressing Diva's like Dana International and Conchita Wurst.

Of course, you may be gender fluid, a mix of these or none. It might all be so new that you do not know quite how you feel about feminization. Perhaps you just want to find out what might be possible. It's okay to be curious. In this book you will discover all about how to make up your face and style your hair. You will find out what you look like as a female version of you from the neck up. If you want to find out about dressing and other things from the neck down read the sister volume to this one: *How to Feminize your Body*.

Finding your look

Right then, having got all that out of the way let's start with the basics. A look is simply defined as the appearance of someone or something at a particular time. Other words are fashion, style, or a way of doing things that is considered acceptable. If you do not have a look yet read through the pages in this book to get some ideas. Scan women's fashion mags and social media, search google, or Pinterest to find styles. Make a scrap book of the things that you and your inner girl like. Find out what is hot and what is not. All women have a certain something. Which means not just style but also pep, vitality, or spirit. What's yours?

Are you refined, ditsy, sophisticated, sweet, delightful, cute, edgy or something else? Perhaps you are into a scene like Steampunk, Bondage, Goth, Cosplay or Japanese Lolita inspired by Anime and Manga comics and want to perfect your look for that. Maybe you are more retro or burlesque or like a 1950s, 1960s, or 1970s look. Each of these genres have their own specifics for makeup, styling, and behaviour (see resources at the back of the book). For example, Goth is very heavy black mascara, dark lipstick and a pale look. In Anime the emphasis is on bigger eyes and long or odango hair to make you look adorable and cute. In a retro style you might want big hair and a particular use of eyeliner or lipstick to match the clothing style of the time, like that iconic 1960s Mary Quant look or another fashion designer. Perhaps you want to copy a Hollywood starlet like Marilyn Monroe, Marlene Dietrich, Sophia Loren, or Bridget Bardot, or go for the Bombshell or Sex Kitten look with loosely waved hair and dramatic eye wings. Maybe you are Maybelline or want that London look.

Once you know the styles, type of makeup and skin tones used to get your look it is much easier to order things online, buy from the local cosmetics shop, or purchase appropriate hair pieces. In the long run this will save you significant amounts of money in wasted materials. You will also learn the vocabulary required to understand the different styles explained in countless web pages and women's magazines. And, of course, be able to girl talk knowledgeably to your girlfriends or women at the makeup counter about fashion and the latest looks. Nothing more embarrassing than going into a shop and realising that you have no idea what to ask for or what the various options mean. That is one of the biggest tells you can give as a crossdresser.

Later we will give you some shopping lists but part of feeling femme is having that interaction and giving voice to your inner girl. Whether it is a real makeover or a trip to the mall you will feel so much more satisfied when you get to act out as a girl. If you are a first timer and/or too shy to go out dressed to buy cosmetics you can always say it is a gift for a female friend. You will find that most beauticians or cosmetic salespeople (which are mostly women) will be enthusiastic about getting all the right stuff for her. You may think that this will all be easier (less embarrassing) online but unless you know what you are buying that can be harder.

It is also useful to get some face to face advice about skin tones and try some before you buy. Products always look different on the face compared to the palette or bottle. There are a few crossdressing boutiques that will take you for a consult, do your makeup, or run classes if a regular shop is too much for you. Check out your local on-line resources or those in a nearby city. The latter is a good idea if you are from a small community and are worried about being recognised. Make a day or a weekend of it. Get to know your girl self.

The four-step method

A good thing to learn is the process (or workflow) of putting on your face. If you study a little art, then you may know that there are several ways to paint a canvas – the so-called indirect and direct methods. Female makeup is a more direct method where after a little priming of the canvas the eye and lip make up is applied direct. Crossdressing or Tgirl makeup uses an indirect method where we spend some time hiding male features before then moving onto the direct method.

No matter what your style or look the sequence is the same. For a female face there are three steps and for a transgendered or male face there are four.

Step 0: is preparing your face by hiding your male attributes. We will have lots more on this in later chapters but basically this involves using skin tones to create a softer face, moving or thinning your eyebrows, and hiding any indication of 5 O'clock shadow. For this step you might need some theatrical or specific crossdressing supplies.

Step 1: here you apply a foundation (to give a smooth skin tone), and concealer (to fill in wrinkles, cover spots, or other blemishes). This creates a background to build the rest of your look and prepares for all the detailed work. You can think of it as blocking in all the initial flesh colour in a portrait painting.

Step 2: is when you start applying the makeup proper. There are three parts to this: blushers, bronzers, and highlighters to create contour and define your cheeks, lipstick to do the same with your mouth and lips, and eye shadow and liner. You might also use a fixer to stop the material rubbing off or smudging and highlights to bring out certain features. The balance and/or style of application of these products is what makes different looks.

Step 3: is all about hair styling. For a woman with an established hair length and style this might involve curling, combing, pinning, and adding accessories like ribbons, clips, or bands. You might want to give your hair extra volume with extensions or use a wig to get the look you want. Wigs can be styled too so the right one can be super versatile. And, of course, you can have different colours and cuts to suit your mood and experiment with being a blonde, brunette, or redhead. It is so much fun being a girl.

Your hair pieces will make you look instantly more femme. But don't rush. Always do the hair last. A woman will pin her hair back or use a wig cap to keep long strands out of the way and avoid sticking them to her face or getting products on the hairs during the early stages. Likewise, it is best to do the whole process in lingerie or at least before you dress otherwise you can mess up your clothes. And, anyway, it is nice to set the mood and feel smooth, silky, and delicate while you femme-up.

Virtual Makeovers

One way to accelerate your learning is to take a virtual makeover. A virtual makeover platform will allow you to experiment with different looks. You can choose from celebrities and models to apply their look to your photo or borrow their hair style. You can do this for free on the web sites of just about any of the big name cosmetic or hair product companies (see resources). The idea is that you can find out what works for you before you buy (hopefully their) products. This can be great fun and will help you decide exactly what styles work for you.

In a virtual makeover you upload a good quality (well lit, non-blurry, no glasses, no makeup etc) passport size picture of yourself and the makeover tool allows you to try on different make up colours, hair pieces, and accessories. Sometimes the app will take your picture using your phone camera or your laptop webcam. They work better if your face is clear of hair and has good contrast. If your hair is short no problem but if you have longer hair pull it back, pin it, or put on a wig cap before you take your picture so that the hair pieces you choose overlay your face properly. Check out the terms and conditions to make sure that your works of art are not included in the public galleries. Some makeup artists or the more extrovert like to show their creations. The default is usually not to include but you may need to tick a box. Often, they just keep your pic for 30 days and then delete it. Anyways, better safe than sorry.

If you find a look or two that you like save the picture on your local device so you can use it as a reference when you do makeup and styling for real. Alternatively, show your sympathetic partner or sign up for a real makeover service. In the former you can have fun together socialising and learning makeup techniques from her to get your look right. Use the tool together to develop your look. For a makeover visit just email or message them your made-up photo when you book and ask them if they can do that style for you on the day.

Sometimes you will find that makeover providers have been to beauty school or have done a theatrical makeup class. If you don't say or know what you want, you may end up looking more drag-queen. That is okay if you just want the experience but can be annoying when you have a look in mind. The better makeover providers are also makeup artists and will be able to do any look you want. For example, they may do bridal hair and makeup, prom or pageant style, period drama hair or the latest celebrity looks. If you are stuck for a choice just say you want an everyday look. That will be good for selfies, blogs, and webpages.

Before you dive into all this, though, here is a warning. It is truly addictive. You will find that there are many ways you can feminize your face and you will fall in and out of love with each one. You might even find that the look you had in mind does not work but discover something else that surprises you. One thing you will definitely learn is just how much hair style and colour can change your appearance. When your face comes together with your hair there will be a magic moment. A ping in the back of your head that says – yes, that's the girl in me. You might feel suddenly overwhelmed and want to cry. Don't smudge your mascara, sweetie.

More ways to express your inner girl

As if you need them here are three more reasons why people get into hair and makeup. Some may sound a little out there, but they cover the whole gamut of people that enjoy feminization. As they say different strokes for different folks.

<u>Couples Play:</u> in this case a female partner may enjoy dressing with you and doing makeup together. The first time this might happen is if you like fancy dress or cosplay. A convention or a Halloween party is the ideal time to femme up. The world is your oyster with this. Costume hire places do all sorts of short fairy tale and sissy outfits such as French maid, Cheerleader, sexy Alice, or Bo peep, or you can just borrow something like a classy evening gown, party, or cocktail dress. People are less likely to question your choice of outfit at a party or a themed convention and some may even comment on how good you look as a girl.

Sometimes it can be a flatmate or long-standing female friend that convinces you to let her do your make up and then dress you. A surprising number of women are curious about male to female transformation. It is an extension to the way they played with dollies when they were growing up. If you get a passable look she will be happy to go out with you to clubs and other venues. Often, she will dress identically as a point of interest. Popular themes are sisters or girlfriends. In short, some women just get a kick out of feminizing guys.

You may also find that if your secret comes out a partner is more tolerant if your dressing stays private and in the bedroom. Or is prepared to turn a blind eye if you do it elsewhere (like a weekend away). This is especially true if you have children. A related type of activity though is cuckolding where a female partner wants a more open relationship. It may be the way she accepts your desires to dress. After all, if you are going to be a girl, she still has needs. If you like this type of thing, it can lead to being dressed and made up while she 'entertains' her male friends. You might be encouraged to watch, play the role of fluffer, or more. Not for everyone but certainly a choice.

Fantasy (or 'forced') Feminization: another reason that you might be interested in makeup and hair styling is because you are being feminized by a partner or a mistress. Forced feminization refers to a male fantasy about being made or 'forced' to dress and adopt female ways. In a female led relationship you might be expected to play the role of wife or maid or something else that requires dressing and doing makeup. This is quite popular amongst the crossdressing community and has very specific requirements. Usually there is some humiliation or embarrassment involved but the male enjoys these sensations and is a willing participant. Nothing is coercive or non-consensual even if it looks like it from the outside. If you find yourself in the latter kind of relationship, leave, seek help and/or contact the authorities.

We are not going to spend a lot of time on the what, why, and how of this specialism other than to note that your significant other will have an idea of how she wants you to look. She may do your face initially to show you what she wants or sit with you until you become proficient but then expect you to do it yourself. Indeed, your partner may give you this book so you can learn how to feminize yourself. This, of course, is intended to socialise you into female ways. You may be required to dress and put on your face at weekends or when you come home from work. She may want you to look pretty for social events with her friends or other like-minded females.

In this genre dressing, nails, makeup and hair are all sources of disciplinary fun. You should expect to be inspected regularly to make sure everything is in tip-top condition and be disciplined according for any errors or omissions. Excessive neatness is the thing. Consequently, you will need to check your makeup and hair as well as other things frequently and spend time touching up as necessary. This book will give you all the tricks and tips you need to meet your partner's requirements. You may also come to appreciate the psychology of why she styles her own hair and makeup in a certain way.

Camming and Skype: if you feminize for social reasons another reason for wanting to perfect your face is camming or skyping with friends. There are many many crossdressing, TV, Tgirl, or Sissy forums or chat rooms where you can video chat or swap details so you can skype more privately. Obviously, always stay safe when you do this. Don't give too many details out and think about what your camera is pointed at over your shoulder. It is surprising what you can see from that little lens into a person's home. Some apps now allow you to blur the background but that is just going to put more emphasis on the detail of your face and hair.

Think about where you place your camera or laptop. If the light is above or behind you it will cast long shadows on your face. If it is a desk light it will uplight giving you that spooky look. Also, you will find that using the built-in camera above your laptop screen will tend to pick out your more angular features. So even if you pay attention to femme makeup you might still look more male. Likewise, depending on the warmth (yellowness) or coolness (bluishness) of your lighting your skin might appear sallow or pale. This can be made worse by heavier makeup which can sometimes be shiny if you don't fix it properly. Conversely, if the lighting is subdued that will hide your features and you will need to do slightly heavier makeup to get your femme look to show up.

To avoid that Boris Karloff look, get a camera that plugs into your device and place it to the side, level or slightly above your face. This will make the best of your features and show off some of your curvy profile and hair. A three-quarter look, or slightly to the front and side, is a popular modelling shot. Obviously, you will need to pay more attention to clothing but, hey, that's a good thing. You will also find that when people can see more of you there is less focus on the detail of your face and they will accommodate your appearance. This means they will adjust to what their brain tells them they are looking at. So, if you are in a nice dress or matching ensemble with long or accessorised hair suddenly your face will look more girly and any flaws in your makeup will not show as much.

About the book

Now, for ease of reading the book is divided into three parts each with a specific purpose. In Part 1 we look at facial structure, consider what makes a face appear male or female, and the types of corrective surgery available. We also get you equipped with all the products and accessories needed to make up your face. Prettiness and delicacy are very subjective, but we will look at what generally makes a face attractive. A large part of this is the configuration or relationship between various elements of your face. How you design your features to meet these stereotypes about cute, adorable, and feminine faces is important to your look but always remember that:

Beauty Attracts the Eye but Personality Captures the Heart

In Part 2 we consider all the techniques you need to mask your most male attributes, make up your eyes and mouth, and ways to contour your face so that it looks softer and more feminine. We use the information in Part 1 to work with your face type and produce a softer female version. We will call this your girl face for easy reference.

Part 3 is all about hair and hair styling. We cover the different types of hair pieces like wigs and extensions and look at different hair styles and accessories. After that we take a tongue-in-cheek but nevertheless useful look at what hair says about your girl personality and include some helpful tricks and tips for the more mature dresser.

The material is laid out in this way so that one technique leads logically onto the next. There are many variations possible and you will find that in the literature other authors do things differently. For example, doing the eyes and mouth before the concealer stage or doing hair before eyes and so on. Generally, though, if you dress before makeup or do hair before makeup you are more likely to smudge or get product on your clothes or in your hair. Use whatever approach works for you. Take the ideas you need and work them into your established routine. If you don't have a process yet copy this one and then fine tune as you learn.

Doing your face and hair can be challenging but also enormous fun. Experiment! Try new looks and flip through magazines or on-line to find things you like. That is all part of your socialization as a girl. Embrace it. You will feel so much more at-ease with yourself, even if your feminization is just a hobby or a naughty indulgence. Make sure you put aside some time for makeup and hair styling as well as just dressing. You can go light (or make-and-go) or spend a morning or afternoon on the detail so that you look the part when you go out, skype, or whatever. The swish of hair about your face or an earring by your cheek will add to your feelings of femininity. It is amazing how much just knowing you have a femme face will boost your confidence. And, your inner girl will feel more able to come out and be herself.

Finally, in picking up a book like this it is likely that you have dabbled with makeup and hair before or thought about it a lot. This means that you may have some specific issues for which you need a solution. Each chapter is more or less self-contained so you can jump to the key issue relevant to you. In each case several options are given so simply choose the one you like the most, are more able to succeed with, or that you want to practice. Although we would love to be able to teleport you to the final look a lot of the techniques require practice. So, if you are a newbie, little steps are best. Please do not get frustrated if you don't turn into a princess first time. Practice makes perfect. That does not mean that learning cannot be fun though – so do immerse yourself in the lovely world that is hair and makeup.

Chapter 2 How femme is your face

In this chapter we compare the anatomy of the male and female face and try to define what it is that people look for in an attractive face. Studying anatomy might sound a big yawn but stick with it because you will get some deep insights into how to be more successful with your makeup. If you are eager to get to more practical things skip on to the next chapter. You can always come back.

Once we have an understanding of the differences between males and females, we will look at the transgendered face. That is, what the effects of hormone therapy can do to give you more feminine looks. And, if you decide, after applying all the techniques in this book, that you need to change some fundamentals of your face we will consider the types of cosmetic surgery that are available.

After that we will turn to the idea of beauty and how the face boffins have tried to define formulas for the ideal face. We'll look at the basic positioning of the elements on your face to show what is considered an archetypal pretty female face. Of course, there are lots of variations and beauty is very subjective but this will give you something to aim for when you start to make up your own face.

How Male and Female heads differ

Forensic scientists can take a human skull add in what they know about muscle groups and fat thickness to reconstruct a person's face and get a good match. That is amazing, but just imagine if you knew what things made you look more male and the ones that made you more feminine. An understanding of what lies under your skin (aka muscle, bone, cartilage, and fat) will give you insights into what you need to do with makeup and accessories.

There are at least six major differences between the skull of an adult human male and female. These are shown in Figure 1 for easy reference and can be listed as follows:

The cranial mass is squarer shaped and bigger in a man. Females are smaller and rounder and the head tapers towards the top. This means that a female face tends to be more oval shaped.

The cranial mass is also deeper front to back than for females. This means that the male forehead tends to slope back more than the female which is more vertical. As a result, the brow ridge or how your forehead joins with the rest of the face can be more obvious.

The supraorbital margin (or outside of the eye socket) is more defined in the female. This means men have more rectangular shaped eye sockets while women have rounder ones. Although the male sockets can be physically bigger the female due to the overall size difference of the skull and the configuration of the various elements means that females can appear to have bigger rounder eyes.

The Zygomatic bone (or cheek bone) is bigger/wider and more obvious in the man. This means that the male face looks squarer and the muscles hang off it to give a flat plane to the cheek. In the woman the bone is shorter and protrudes more at the front. Leaner muscles give the cheek bone more definition to create the so-called apple. The apple often appears more reddish after exercise or excitement because the thinner skin shows more blood circulation. Colour here can give you a fresh faced or healthy look.

The mandible (or Jaw bone) is more square in the male compared to the female. The angle of the jaw from the ear to the chin is slightly less in the female. At the front, the jaw is wider in the man and tapers more to a point in the female. This gives men a squarer thicker set lower face with a wider chin. Females on the other hand are softer and tend to have smaller chins. The thickness of the muscle that holds the mandible to the skull is also bigger in a man than a woman which gives the impression of a stronger bunched jaw compared to a softer female jaw.

The supercilary arch (or bit that connects your forehead to the front of your face) is more pronounced in the male than the female. This means that men tend to have a brow ridge which, if very prominent, can look a bit stone age. The depression at the top of your nose can also be deeper than the equivalent female.

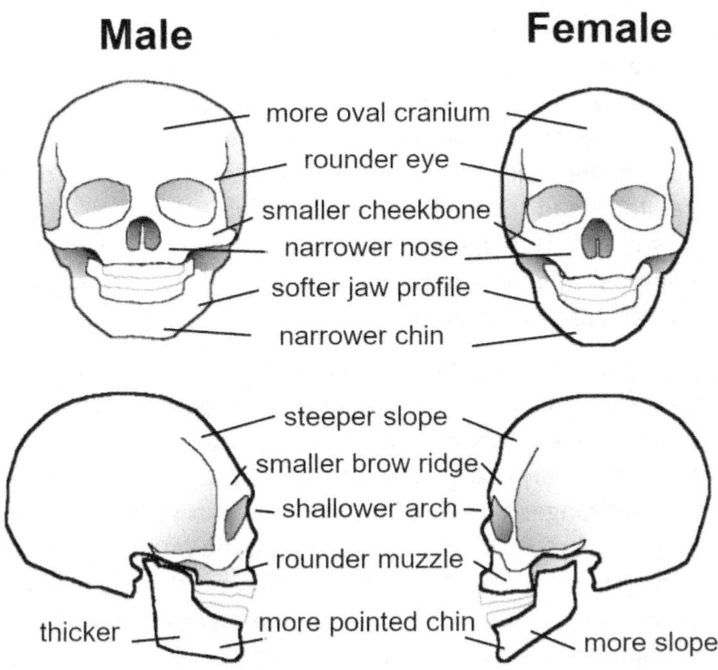

Figure 1 Differences between male and female heads

The effects of muscle and skin

Given the above structure the details of your face emerge from how the muscles and cartilage attach to these bones. Depending on how thick your muscles are and how much fat you carry, the face will have more or less definition. As a rule, females tend to have less (leaner) muscle mass over all than males. Once the muscles are in place the skin is then supported by a layer of fat. The fat can be of different depths depending on where it is. So, for example, the forehead has very little fat while the cheeks have more. Generally, females have more fat under their skin (so called subcutaneous fat) than men so their features are more rounded as a result.

Figure 2 gives you a map of the major muscle groups and planes (or angles) of the face. The planes will be important when we get to contouring in Part 2. Putting all this together we can observe the following visible differences between male and female faces.

Hair line: because of the slope of the cranium the male hair line tends to have a rounded M shape. This gets more pronounced as men age and testosterone levels drop and hair recedes (so-called pattern baldness). It can start at any age and some men just have more pronounced M shapes than others. Male hairstyles also tend to play on this feature. Women on the other hand have a straighter hair line across the more vertical forehead. Sometimes there is a V-shape at the centre (a widow's peak). This means that some female faces can appear more heart shaped. Men can have one too with a less pronounced M which softens the upper face a little.

Eyebrows: the more defined brow ridge means that male eyebrows appear closer to the eyes. Female ones appear higher on the brow. Muscles in this area allow you to pull your eyebrows up or down in the centre to show surprise or concern. Male eyebrows do tend to be a little bushier and longer than female ones and can sometimes meet in the middle (monobrow). Also they run around the outside of the eye socket to frame the eye more. But generally, there isn't that much difference except of course that women shape and style their brows more than men. Whatever the current fashion trend female brows can be thinner or thicker. More on that later.

Eye Levels: the difference in the eye sockets mean that the upper and lower eyelids can be attached slightly differently to the muscle and bone. The eye operates like a small slit in the skin and muscle (orbicularis oculi) laid over the eyeball. When the skin is pulled back by tensing of the muscles the eye opens and when the muscles relax it closes. The slit in Males is more or less horizontal on the face. In females it can be horizontal or slant upwards or downwards towards the nose.

This tilting gives the eye a more cat like appearance which some people find attractive.

Lips: the mouth is another slit in the skin and muscle (orbicularis oris). The principle though is the same when the muscles are pulled or relaxed the slit opens or closes. And, of course, when we open our jaw, we can stretch the opening wider. The whole arrangement of the muscles around the mouth and lips is referred to as the muzzle. It is gently rounded following the curve of the upper teeth. Because this area is narrow and more curved in females, they tend to have a more pronounced muzzle. The mouth is also a little smaller than in the man. The lips are fuller. The upper male lip is thinner and flatter and there is more distance between it and the nose – hence the phrase keeping a stiff upper lip when referring to being brave or manly.

Cheeks: we already mentioned the apple of the cheek as a point of distinction, but the cheek bone is also where the muscles that control the muzzle are attached. They allow you to smile by pulling the corner of the muzzle upwards. There are several muscles for this job and depending on how lean they are or how much fat is on the cheek they can leave gaps when operated. Hence a person may dimple when they smile or laugh. Because females have leaner muscles and the muzzle is more defined this is more likely. Also, there is a joining point of all these muscles called the node just to the side of the mouth. You might also get a little quirk at this point when you smirk or smile.

Nose: the nose is mainly skin over cartilage which defines the openings of the nostrils. There is a pad at the end which is called the ball of the nose. Because the overall dimensions of the female head are smaller, females tend to have smaller and more narrow noses. The ball is often smaller, rounder and a little flatter giving the cute button nose look but not always. Usually the end of the female nose turns up a little so more of the join between the nostrils is visible. A further set of muscles run up the side of the nose which allow you to corrugate (or wrinkle) your nose (and pull you eyebrows down) this together with muscles attached to the chin of the jaw allow you to frown. Nose cartilage continues to grow (slowly) throughout your lifetime so your nose will get bigger as you age.

Jaw and chin: the mandible is not attached directly to the skull. It depends on a strong muscle (the Masseter) at the sides which acts like a rubber band to keep it in place and to allow the mouth to open and close. Because the male jawbone is bigger and heavier the muscle is larger which gives more jaw definition. The lower half of the muzzle is connected to the chin. These muscles allow you to frown but there is also a muscle on the tip called the mentalis (the pouting muscle). This muscle splits into two branches going to each side of the lower lip. Depending on how much fat there is over it or how lean it is you might see a cleft (or dimple) in the chin.

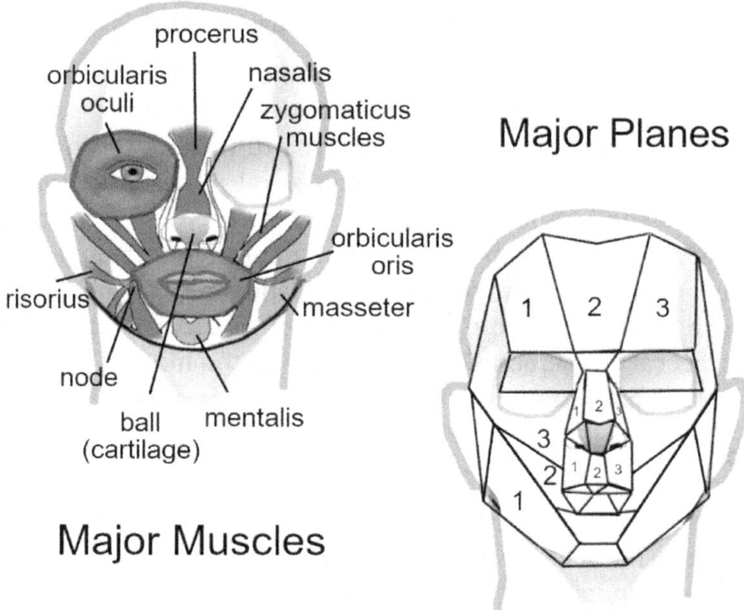

Figure 2 Muscles and Planes of the Face

The Transgendered Face

The previous sections have made comparisons for the extremes of maleness and femaleness. Actually, everyone has a slightly different skull and muscle configuration. The sizes, shape, and length of the bones in the skull as well as the attachment and length of the muscles all vary. An interesting, if not entirely helpful question, is when does a face stop being male and become female. Everyone is on this spectrum between male and female. So, we all have transgendered faces to some degree or another.

People generally fall into a small number of body types. If you have read the sister volume to this one on *Feminizing your Body,* you'll recall that the extremes of the manly man and the girly girl account for only something like 10% of the population. The most common body type (about 40% of the population) is a rectangle or straight up and down shape. There is no reason to think that faces don't follow a similar pattern. The chances are that if your frame size is small or towards the middle or female end of the body type spectrum you will also have some femme face features.

Usually though we refer to a transgendered face as one belonging to an individual who is assigned one sex at birth and undergoes hormone replacement therapy to look more like their chosen gender. In our case this is a male transitioning to female. Hormone therapy controls or reduces testosterone and increases estrogen. Estrogen is the female hormone that influences breast development, fat distribution, and the size of muscles in the body. Women tend to have fat distributed on the butt, hips, and breasts but also all over the body including the face. Testosterone is the male hormone and concentrates fat more on the torso and not on the face or limbs.

A person in transition will change the balance of these chemicals in the body and this (over time) will redistribute fat and slim down muscles. The face will get softer as a result. This will help disguise the square features of the male skull but won't take them away completely. Hormone replacement doesn't affect bone structure at all or for that matter how your muscles have attached themselves to your skull. But they do affect the size and shape of the contours under your skin which influences how light will reflect off the planes of your face. These factors can make you appear more feminine.

It might be useful to check yourself out right now by feeling the bones and playing with the muscles in your face. How male are you? And how female are you? Take a note of your most male features so that you can check them off as we get around to feminizing your face.

How many female features do you have already? Tally them up. If you have more female features than male ones you have a female face. The more femme characteristics you have the easier it is going to be to get a passable look when we do makeup and other things.

Facial Feminization Surgery

Okay so you can get a softer face as a result of hormone therapy but what if that isn't enough. Well there are some standard cosmetic surgery procedures that will help. Given our list above it will not be a surprise that these are predominantly confined to the upper third of the face. There are some lower face options as well. Here is a list:

Brow lift: as the name suggests because a man's eyebrows are usually below the brow ridge and a woman's are above or on the brow ridge this procedure lifts the eyebrows to the female position. The bone on the brow ridge might also be shaved down for a reduced profile.

Orbit Recontouring: as we indicated the outer female eye socket has a slightly different shape with more angled outer edges. They also narrow towards the nose. So this procedure attempts to sculpt the eye orbit for a more female look. This will affect the way the eyelids frame the eye.

Rhinoplasty (or the nose job): attempts to reduce the nose and reshape it by removing bone and cartilage. The male nose is a little longer and wider than the female version. In a female nose the ball of the nose is smaller and makes the tip point up a little. This sounds great but there are all sorts of problems that can arise from the nose job and it can ruin your face when it goes badly. The major problem is the nostrils closing or narrowing so that it is hard to breathe, or your voice sounds nasally like you have a heavy cold. The latter might make your voice sound deeper or more male.

Lip Augmentation: this procedure has two functions. First is to contour the upper muzzle area between the nose and the mouth which is often longer in males than females. And as we noted the upper lip is wider and thinner, so this is reduced and plumped up. Ideally, for the best female look, the incisor teeth should be slightly visible when your mouth is open and relaxed. To fix the mouth a wedge of skin is removed just below the nose which pulls the lip upwards. Bits from the edges of the upper lip are also taken which pulls it inwards for a smaller fuller look. Additional filling may be used to plump the upper and lower lips. Injectable fillers tend to last about six months. Using your own fat is possible but can be reabsorbed by the body. Many people say that changing your mouth has the biggest effect on feminizing your face but we also know of many horror stories where lip plumping goes terribly wrong. Cheaper is not always best in this regard. Later we will show you some non-surgical tricks to get the appearance of a smaller fuller mouth.

Cheek Implants: the female cheek bone is smaller and has more projection, so the objective here is to remove bone and restructure the cheek for a more female appearance. An implant is often added which creates the 'apple' or one is rebuilt from fatty tissue elsewhere on the body. An implant can slip or dislodge which could give you a lopsided appearance. And, on rare occasions granulomas can form as your immune system reacts to inflammation or foreign objects in your face that it cannot eliminate.

Chin and Jaw contouring: as the name suggests this reshapes the chin to make it smaller and adjusts the back of the jaw to make it less square. Since the jaw is longer in the male a section of bone is removed to shorten it. The masseter (or chewing muscle) can also be reduced to make the jaw profile narrower. Male chins are squarer so the bone can be shaved down to give a more rounded appearance. Because the chin and cheek support the muscles to the muzzle these two procedures are often done together.

Facial hair removal: another point to note is that you will likely carry more facial hair than the average female. Depending on the level of growth you will have to shave regularly maybe even daily. If the hair is darker it will be a challenge to hide. And, even if you shave close it will mean that your girl time is limited because the hair will grow back during the day. The infamous 5 O'clock shadow. We will give you ways to hide this male feature in Part 2 but if you are a regular or 24/7 girl you might want to the think about having the hair removed permanently. Modern cosmetic procedures like laser or electrolysis can be used. The latter is more effective if your facial hair is light coloured or thin. It can take up to six months to say goodbye to all this hair but after that you will have a smooth face and can dispense with makeup procedures designed to hide your shadow.

You may be tempted by surgical intervention because it can complete you as a person. And knowing that your bone structure is more female can be psychologically satisfying. However, all of these procedures are close to vital sense organs and the musculature, blood supply, and nerves are all very intricate. Any major problems such as infection, immune system responses, movement of implants, or even nicking a nerve in the process make these procedures very risky. You don't want to end up having to live with a lifelong complication or a lopsided face. Other procedures like butt lifts or a boob job can also go wrong but at least you can cover them up. A mistake on your face is almost impossible to hide. That all sounds a little scary. We don't want to put you off the idea of surgery completely, but it makes sense to see what can be achieved with clever makeup techniques.

What makes an attractive face?

Did you ever stop to ask yourself why women feel the need to paint their faces and arrange their hair? All this stems from the ideals of attractiveness and beauty which means different things to different people. In fact, it may be that a mix of male and female features can actually make you more attractive. Say, what?

No, really. If you look at women's magazines and the fashion pages, female models with masculine features are not difficult to find. Often the squarer masculine jaw is seen as quite striking on the female (it is still softer of course). Slightly longer noses are also easy to find. A few years ago, the model, Cara Delevingne, appeared on the scene to massive acclaim. Cara has what could be called a striking boyish look. She was famous for her thicker fuller eyebrows and if you look at her properly, she has a slightly longer nose, thinner wider top lip, and squarish back jaw. She combines that of course with lovely female eyes, rounder cheeks, and a smaller chin.

Sadly, people are not as accepting when it comes to a male face that has effeminate qualities. A study from University of Otago, Warwick Business School, and University of California, San Diego found that male faces with feminine features are attractive in some contexts but not others. The so-called 'Johnny Depp Effect' indicates that many women are attracted to men with female faces. The results seem to be on the basis that males with female faces tend to make good carers and providers (or nice Dads) while traditional male features indicate a bad boy persona but stronger (or better) genes. Generally, though, feminine faces are preferred unless people are forced to pigeonhole a person by gender.

If we indulge ourselves for a moment it is possible to come up with a spectrum of likeability for faces. For example, are you plain, handsome, pretty, statuesque, or cute? The first two hark back to the time of Jane Austen. Are you a plain Jane with nothing disagreeable about your features but nothing remarkable either? The word handsome is now confined mostly to a description of men but in the past it was politely applied to females as well. In the novel, *Pride and Prejudice,* Mr Darcy surprises two sisters who are referring to his love interest, Elizabeth Bennet, as plain by saying she is one of the most handsome women he has met. This implies some striking quality like your eyes, or smile, or something else that marks you out from the crowd.

Of course, we all expect females to be pretty, which means to be attractive in a delicate kind of way but still falling short of being beautiful. Statuesque implies that a woman is tall, graceful, and dignified but also has striking looks which may incorporate that stronger jaw line. Think Greek goddess, like Hera (goddess of women, marriage, and childbirth) or Aphrodite (love, passion, beauty, pleasure and procreation), or even Artemis (hunting and chastity). By the way, Artemis was called Diana in Roman mythology and is the basis for Wonder Woman. She was the only Amazon not to be conceived by a man. And finally, we have the cute look which means to be attractive in a pretty and endearing way. We often apply cute to children and animals but the features of big eyes, small nose, and chin is what usually makes someone cute in looks. More on this later.

If your objective is to be passable then any of these descriptions would be more than adequate. Take a few moments to think about your looks and how you might be classified. What would you be happy with as the result of your makeover? Handsome or plain might work provided you can be accepted as a girl. Do you have a particular girl feature or something pretty about you? With a little help from makeup and styling we can bring those out.

Face metrics

Since the times of antiquity people have tried to come up with a formula to define beauty. Basically, this amounts to looking at the relationship between all the features of a face and deciding what defines the most attractive. If a portrait artist is even slightly off with the positioning of the eyes, nose, and mouth a pretty girl will look less so. Of course, it has a lot to do with facial symmetry. Nobody really thinks Quasimodo is attractive – at least not on the outside.

Let's look at a few ways of measuring a face.

The golden section: the Greeks were famous for the golden section. All their spectacular buildings (like the Parthenon) were built according to this ratio which is supposed to be the most pleasing to the eye. For this reason, it is often called the Divine proportion. And, of course, they couldn't help applying it to bodies and faces. The surprising thing is that it does a remarkably good job of defining exactly why we look the way we do and how attractive a face appears.

The golden section is defined as constant value that is the ratio of two parts of a line segment. Draw a line of any length and then mark a spot to divide it in two. Call the longest part **a** and the shorter part **b**. The golden ratio is simply the value **(a+b)/a** when it equals **a/b**. This occurs only when the ratio reaches the value 1.618033. The Greeks were so impressed with this that they gave it a name, *Phi*. You can easily find the cutting point using *Phi* and the length of the line.

Okay, back to faces. The vertical or horizontal arrangement of many facial features satisfies the golden ratio. Draw a square with the pupils at the upper corners and the lower corners at the ends (nodes) of your mouth. Yes, it will be close to a square on just about everyone. Now find the golden ratio for the horizontal and vertical lines of the square. Guess what. Where you cut the lines will be exactly where the nose appears. If you draw a rectangle around your nose with the inner point of your eyes as the upper corners and the bottom of the nose as the opposite side. The golden ratio tells you where the tip of your nose is positioned. The same applies for the centre of your mouth (or where the mouth slit appears between the top and bottom lip (and, also, where your two front teeth are positioned). If you take half the length (width) of your upper lip and find the ratio this will define the position of the little depression downwards on the top lip. That is often referred to as Cupids Bow (aww!). There are other features that satisfy this relationship too and it is not just confined to your face. But, anyway, you can see why the Greeks thought it was special.

According to the golden section a face (or body) is most attractive when all its features conform to the ratio. Every so often someone applies the numbers to a collection of faces to rate them. The most recent one is due to Dr Julian De Salva who runs The Centre for Advanced Facial Cosmetic and Plastic Surgery in London. His top ten female celebrity faces are: Amber Heard (91.85%), Kim Kardashian (91.39%), Kate Moss (91.06%), Emily Ratajkowski (90.8)%, Kendall Jenner (90.18%), Helen Mirren (89.93%), Scarlett Johansson (89.82%), Selena Gomez (89.57%), Marilyn Monroe (89.41%), and Jennifer Lawrence (89.24%). The percentage is a totalling of how close all their facial features matched the ratio. You might want to work out your own ratios using that virtual makeover pic and see if you have any divine features.

The rule of thirds: a simpler metric is often used by artists to define the proportions of the face and human body. This is called the rule of thirds. The idea is that you split up an image or object by two equally spaced horizontal and two equally spaced vertical lines to form a grid. The places where the lines cross forms a point of interest. If you place an object at a grid point it will often look more appealing than if you put it in the centre. If you think about it that means splitting a line into a third and two thirds. This gives a ratio of 3/2 = 1.5 which is not a million miles away from the golden ratio.

Leonardo Da Vinci used this idea to define a vertical (mid-) line on the face. The first third will reach from your hairline to the brow line. The second third will stretch from the brow line to the nostrils of your nose. The third section will reach from the bottom of the nose to the tip of the chin. Likewise you can define a horizontal line. The first third will go from one ear to the centre of the pupil of the nearest eye. The second third will go from one pupil to the other. And the last third will go from that pupil to the other ear. It gets weirder though. If you divide up the nose, the bottom of your eyes will usually not go lower than a third from the brow. Likewise, the distance from the bottom of the nose to the chin can also be divided into thirds. The top third is the distance from your nose to opening of your mouth. The (closed) mouth covers the middle third. And the bottom third is the chin. Your ears occupy the middle third of your face but out to the side so the top of your ear is close to the brow line and the ear lobe aligned with the bottom of the nose.

Of course, not all people match these criteria exactly some people have a larger forehead, a longer nose, or a small chin area, or a wider face. And, it only applies to adults. Children have slightly different ratios. Most strikingly the lower parts of the face in babies covers half with the other half the forehead. It is only as we grow that the face lengthens to approximate thirds. An adult will be considered cute if they retain some of these 'baby' features because the eyes will appear bigger, the nose more upturned, and chin smaller relative to the rest of the face. Pretty women often have some childlike features. In the past the stereotype for a feminine woman was that she was childlike, dependent and passive. Women have evolved all sorts of makeup tricks to reinforce this observation.

The Five S's: eyes have an important part to play in your feminization. Eyes grab attention and can show attraction and interest. When you look into someone's eyes you can fall in love. They are the windows on your inner girl. Because women spend so much time on their eyes with eye shadow, eyeliner, lashes, and mascara it is worth taking a more detailed look at how eyes can be classified. There are literally hundreds of ways to define an eye. Fortunately, Kendra Powell, a makeup and hair specialist, has reduced it to just five metrics: shape, size, situation, setting and slant. Let's look at each of these.

Shape: female eyes come in two varieties almond or round. This refers to the shape of the slit that forms the opening in the skin to reveal your eye. In an almond eye the slit is shaped like (guess what) an almond this gives it a narrower cat like appearance and can look striking with a downward slant. In a round eye the slit is more circular and may look like a wide lemon shape. Round eyes tend to be straighter (more horizontal) but because of the wider opening they reveal more of your iris and eyeball which make them look bigger. If you can see the iris completely your eyes are round. If the slit covers some of the iris they are almond. The degree of coverage means that you can rate eyes according to roundness.

Size: are your eyes large, small or average. This sounds difficult to judge without looking at other people but is really quite easy. How much space do your eyes take up on your face? A way to measure is to see if the width of one eye is the same, bigger, or smaller than the width of your nose. (that's the rule of thirds). Likewise, is the height of your eye a third of your nose length, or middle third of your face. If your eyes are greater in one or both direction your eyes are large. And if they are smaller in one of both directions your eyes are small.

The size and shape of your eyes determines how much makeup you can use on them without swamping your face or making your eyes look smaller. Remember women appear to have bigger eyes than men.

Situation: describes how the upper eyelid is positioned. Is it a Monolid, Creased, or Hooded? And, how does it fit in the socket, is it deep set or prominent?

A Monolid is what we normally associate with Asian people where the eyelid is a straight connection from the brow to slit. It can be a striking look and there is less difference between men and women so easier to feminize. Most lids though are creased. That means that the skin from brow to slit follows the contour of the eye socket and wraps around the eyeball. Your eye is hooded if the skin above the crease sags or hangs so that it looks as though there isn't a crease. Hooded eyes are seen as attractive in men (a lot of male models have them) but most women hate them because it causes all sorts of issues with doing your eyes. They can also make you look older.

In deep set eyes the eyeball appears further back in the socket so the bunching of skin around the eye slit is more noticeable. One of the reasons for this is a more prominent brow ridge that extends out to sides of your face rather than fading as it does with females. The upper lid can also be more visible between the brow and crease. In prominent eyes the eyeball sticks out of (or protrudes from) the socket. This pushes out the lower lid under the eye which can make your eyes look baggy or swollen. Usually you can see more of the eyelid from the crease to the eye lash. Hooded eyes occur with both these types which may add to the depth or hide the protrusion. You'll need different makeup strategies to feminize these types.

Setting: describes how your eyes are positioned relative to your nose. Are they wide apart, close together, or proportional? If your eyes satisfy the rule of thirds, they are proportional. The distance between your pupils will be the same length as your forehead or your nose, or from nose to chin. If your eyes are close together the distance between the pupils will be less. Tennis players or marksmen often have this look – the theory is that the tighter parallax of the eyes helps them zero in on the ball or target. If your pupils are further apart than the standard your eyes are wide. This gives more space for your nose so it can look wider and/or flatter. Females tend to have narrower noses.

Slant: in relation to the horizontal are your eyes straight, slant downward from the side of your face, or slant upwards. To find out draw a horizontal line from the corner of your inner eye and just below the top of your ears (which occupy the middle third at the side of your head). Now check out the outside corner of your eye slit. If it is above the line your eyes are downward. If it is below the line your eyes are upwards. And, if it is more or less level you have straight eyes. Male eyes are mostly straight, so we want to use eyeliner and other stuff to give you a bit of a tilt.

By the way we are assuming that when you measure your face you are looking straight on like a passport photo. If you don't do this, you may get slightly different answers depending on which side of your face you are measuring because foreshortening of the image will affect the results. For example, you might see more of your iris or the white of your eye if you are looking sideways, up or down. The vertical thirds are also foreshortened if you are looking up or down. You might even get some variations on left and right even when straight on because all faces have a slight (barely noticeable) asymmetry on the midline. This is why people say they have a good and a bad side when it comes to posing for photographs.

The more mature face

The way a young woman and an older one applies makeup and style their hair is different. We can dismiss this as society having different expectations but there are some physiological changes that also mean a different approach is required.

As we age, we deposit more fat around the body and that includes the face. The muscles get tired and stretched from constant use and the skin gets looser, wrinkles, and sags due to gravity. All this means that your facial features get looser as you age. The whole face starts to kind of slide downwards. This makes the jowls that hang on the cheeks and cover the jaw. The softening effect also means you cannot use the same contouring techniques that you can on a younger face. We also tend to develop some puffiness under the eyes creating bags that are slightly discoloured. The skin over the brow line might also sag a little and the upper eyelids may become more hooded.

None of that sounds appealing but there is a whole industry out there to sell you creams that tighten, fill wrinkles, hydrate, and rejuvenate the skin. Use them if you feel the need. Some people also go for the surgery option with a facelift. You can have your eyelids lifted too – a process called Blepharoplasty – to reduce hooding and give you a crease. If you come to feminization later in life, or see the ravages of time approaching, you might also combine a lift with some of the other feminizing procedures we outlined above. Later we will give you some makeup and style tips to help.

Getting Foxy

A few years ago, scientists did an experiment to see how much of an image was required to provoke recognition. Sheep were shown pictures of foxes and their responses analysed to see if it triggered a sense of fear. Remarkably, they found that even a simple line drawing was 'foxy' enough to trigger a sheep's innate wariness. The idea though is that the brain (even a sheep brain) extracts the essential features of a face and classifies it as good or bad. One theory of attractiveness is that we are genetically programmed to react positively both emotionally and sexually to people that meet certain criteria. Just like sheep with foxes. Our prettiness recognition is built in.

Perhaps that is what the golden section and the rule of thirds is all about. Anyway, animators exploit this fact heavily by designing characters that trigger our cuteness response. They do it in a clever way though because to generate an animation requires hours of work drawing the same character in lots of different poses. So, when animators design a character, they slim it down to the essential brush strokes and shapes to get the character's unique quality. Understanding how to do that with your makeup will not only give you that cute look but also reduce your time in front of the makeup mirror.

Check it out for yourself by looking at your favourite Disney princesses or Manga or Anime characters. Ariel (*the little mermaid*) has big round eyes with a bit of a slant and a fuller face. Jasmine (*Aladdin*) has classic almond eyes with a longer nose. Belle (*Beauty and the Beast*) has eyes somewhere in between and a bit straighter but has a small chin and the hint of apples. Cinderella has straighter, roundish eyes, with some cheek definition but a more pouty mouth. Sleeping Beauty as rounder eyes and a slightly upturned nose with a well-defined muzzle and lip area. Snow White has slightly almond eyes but it is all about the red cheeks and the smaller protruding muzzle. Elsa (*Frozen*) has huge eyes which combine almond with round and a very small chin compared to the nose. Anna is very similar (they are sisters) and a little more in proportion but the hair colour and style makes all the difference. See how the hair softens or defines the face. Which one do your think is the most attractive or elegant? Look at the face construction and the placement of the elements and how it meets or breaks the rule of thirds.

Can you see what makes them all cute? Female characters are all foxy looking. And we don't mean sexy necessarily although a lot of them have a certain kind of appeal. Generally, they have overly big eyes, a small nose, the muzzle protrudes, and the chin is a little pointed. Recognise any of that? Now we are not suggesting that you make yourself up like a Disney character – though it might be an idea for a cosplay party. No, the point is that there are only one or two things you need to define to get your own look. Keeping it simple will mean that you can put your face on quickly and reliably every day or whenever you want with the minimum of fuss. Like an animator. Simplify back to the essentials that communicate femininity and avoid over doing your makeup.

And finally …

Okay so hopefully you now have a much better appreciation of the female face and the task facing you when you feminize your own face. If you understand the proportions of male and female faces you will find that the differences on the placement of features is only minor. We can compensate for those differences using makeup. And, with the clever use of the planes of the face we can re-shape what people see to give the illusion of a much more feminine face. If we take account of the stereotypes that people use to process for attractiveness, we can also give you a cute or adorable look. All we need to do is discover your pretty features and enhance them.

A couple of other important things that will contribute to your total look are the neck and ears. Male necks tend to be thicker than female ones and have that very male protrusion the Adam's apple. The neck joins the head to the body and is usually more visible with female clothing. This means that we will have to think about fading in your face makeup to the rest of your skin tone to avoid an obvious tidemark. This is also true for females but they generally have a lighter skin tone on their face to start with. We will use some darker tones to hide facial hair and soften the jaw so we need to keep this in mind. You can, of course, have a procedure, *Chondrolaryngoplasty* (or tracheal shave) to reduce the Adam's apple if it is too obvious or distracting.

We often think that females have more delicate ears than men. Yes, the total ear size is larger in men but the earlobe weight and height are just about the same. Women tend to cover more of their ear with hair so that only the lobe is visible. This means that if you do likewise, you'll already have girly ears and can use earrings and jewellery to help soften your face. More on that in Part 3.

So, to summarize. There is no one single universally attractive face but the cosmetic and makeup industry like to sell us one because it helps them shift products. If we can just feminize your face a little bit you will feel more authentic and get a much more rewarding outcome. Remember, though, that it is your individuality that makes you beautiful and unique. The configuration of the various elements of your face is one of the ways that we define attractiveness. It appears that the body follows some simple rules as to where it builds features on your face. We looked at various criteria, the golden section, the rule of thirds, and the 5 S's for eyes. The important takeaway from this is that faces vary around these ideal proportions. If you start enumerating all the ways the various elements can align themselves, you end up with the wide variety of faces we see in real life. Just nudging your features in the right direction will instantly make you look more pretty and femme.

Chapter 3 Getting Equipped

This chapter is all about the things you need to start your journey into cosmetics. We will look at the different types of products on the market and identify the essentials from the nice-to-have. At the end we will put together a shopping list so that you can get equipped and be ready to start the practical process of putting on your face.

We will cover four things: products for your face, eyes, and lips; applicators to get the product onto and off your face; accessories that make the job easier; and a few tips on how to use your new tools. It helps in this regard to think like an artist getting ready to paint a canvas except the work of art is three dimensional not flat and two-dimensional. To cut all this information down to a manageable size we are not going to get involved with choosing colours. We will get to all that later and if you have done a virtual makeover or built your scrapbook of looks you probably have some ideas already.

Even if you know your colours for things like lipstick and eyeshadow there are still different types of products you can use. Just like an artist can choose from pastels, or watercolours, or oils and may be good with one medium but not another you will find that you have a preference or find it easier to work your magic with one kind of product or applicator than another. This all takes time and experimentation to discover and master so let's start at the beginning.

A brief history of cosmetics (or makeup)

Even as far back as the Greeks and Romans women used white (lead) powder to lighten their complexion. A light skin tone was preferred because it didn't make you look sun tanned. That's ironic given the modern-day obsession with tanning products. But originally it indicated that you didn't have to work in the fields and so had high status. Helen of Troy – the face that launched a thousand ships – in Greek legend, was noted for her pale and milky complexion. Today the reverse is true. In most cities people work indoors in unnatural light and look pasty. A suntan makes you look healthy and indicates that you have enough leisure time to enjoy life which is another indicator of status.

Our ancient ancestors also knew that an attractive face shows youth and vitality. Powder could be used to cover over blemishes and wrinkles. A pinch on the (apple of the) cheek or a bit of rouge could give you a rosy glow. And biting on a cherry or a strawberry or some such fruit could make your lips look red and glossy. All these attributes are indicators of good blood circulation and health. And, of course, when it comes to finding a mate facial symmetry and big docile (or doe) eyes were considered attractive qualities. So nicely shaped eyebrows, full fluttery lashes, and bigger pupils were all things a woman wanted.

We have the Egyptians to thank for all that black mascara and thicker eyelashes. You can see this thick eyeliner in hieroglyphics and on golden statutes of goddesses and royal families. They used kohl made from stibnite. The modern equivalent is ground charcoal. The cleopatra look was popular in the 1960s – think Elizabeth Taylor, who played the part in the epic film or if you like a bit of kitsch, Amanda Barry, who placed the role in the parody, *Carry on Cleo*. During the renaissance (14th-16th centuries) fashionable women drank the juice of Belladonna, or deadly nightshade, to dilate their pupils and redden the skin. Belladonna means beautiful lady in Italian, but the plant is also highly poisonous and was often the assassin's choice because it could be slipped easily into food or drink. Some women died from taking too much. Below we'll show you some safe ways to do the same thing as those renaissance beauties.

The modern-day obsession with makeup though has Hollywood to thank. In 1904, Max Factor moved his family and business to

California where he became the biggest distributor of made-to-order wigs and theatrical makeup to the developing film industry. Traditionally, grease paint had been used in theatres for stage makeup and applied using a stick of product. But when it was used for films the colours did not look right and it could not be applied thinly enough. Max Factor perfected a new 'powder' product that wasn't so greasy and was very adaptable. Soon many of the Hollywood actresses of the time were visiting his beauty salon to have their face done.

By 1918, he had developed the Colour Harmony range which allowed him to customise makeup to different people using a range of skin tones. He also developed different exaggerations of the lips to make actresses distinctive in their looks. By 1920 he was referring to his technique and products as makeup. Previously, women in polite society referred to these things as cosmetics. The term makeup was seen as vulgar and something confined to the stage or dubious people. Eventually though the term stuck and he started to make his own brand products.

When Technicolor films became the new thing, Max developed a product known as Pancake. The problem with the old products was that it left a sheen on the skin which reflected too much in the camera. This new product was so good that women on the sets started stealing it to use privately. But it was too dark to be used for evening outings with subdued lighting. Eventually they began to make lighter shades and realised the commercial possibilities and the rest as they say is history.

Altogether the company Max founded made over nineteen innovations which are in most cosmetic products today. We can thank him not just for face powders but also lip gloss, nail polish, smear proof and waterproof products as well as the first concealer. So more than anyone crossdressers owe him a big thank you.

Basic Products

The first set of products we need are all intended to give the face a nice uniform tone and smoothness. We have primers, foundation, and concealer. Normally they are applied to the face in that order but in feminization we have two concealer stages one after the primer and one after the foundation. Here is what they do:

Primer: if you have ever done any decorating or painted a wall, you will appreciate the need for the primer. Basically, it fills some imperfections and seals the surface. This stops the following product layers from soaking into the skin or clogging in wrinkles, fine lines, and large pores. Our skin contains oils which can soak up through the makeup and spoil the look. So basically, the primer helps your other makeup go on easier and last for longer. If you have beautiful skin that isn't that oily you might not need to prime. Men though tend to have more oily skin than women.

Foundation: comes in a cream or powder form and is applied to the face to give it a uniform colour. It also allows you to change the overall skin tone (making it lighter or darker). Some foundations also act as a moisturiser or a sunscreen or even an astringent (to tighten up skin). A BB cream is a lighter type of foundation with some of the above features. A CC (or colour correcting) cream is a foundation that will correct for red patches or sallow colour on your face. They do this by containing light diffusing particles.

Concealers: are also colour correctors but are used to mask dark circles, age spots, large pores, and other small blemishes visible on the skin. They are like foundation only thicker to hide stronger pigments by blending into the surrounding skin tone. You use the concealer after the foundation so that you use less product. The foundation covers lots of little imperfections and the concealer the big ones. In feminization we also use concealer before the foundation to mask 5 O'clock shadow and to hide bits of the eyebrows that are characteristic of the male face (see Part 2).

Products for Contouring

The next three things you need are Blush, Highlighter, and Bronzer. These products allow you to define more detail or contour your face from the uniform colour of the foundation.

Blush: as the name suggests is used to give you a healthier looking complexion. It adds a little glow to your skin that gives a more youthful appearance. Reddish powder blush is used to give those apples a little extra pep. A cream blush can give you shiny skin. You have to be careful applying blush because subtle shades are more effective than garish ones. A lot of people get this wrong and that's when they start to look like a doll, a clown, or the sugar plum fairy.

Highlighter: is a product that reflects light. The main use is for contouring to brighten the skin. A lighter skin tone can often give an area more focus or create the illusion of height by creating depth and angles on the skin. We'll look at highlighting and depth using the planes of the face in Part 2.

Bronzer: does what it indicates which is to tan or darken the skin. So again, it can make you look healthy but in a different way to blush. Bronzer is also used to darken skin without masking it. Darker values add warmth and depth and make your skin look rounder and more curved but it can also be used for a dramatic look by creating sharper or more angular features.

The art to feminizing your face is contouring and this means that you use the foundation as a base colour and then use lighter and darker tones to give depth and roundness to your features.

Fixers and Finishers

The last thing you need for the general face is a way to keep your product in place. Here we have two possible products Fixers and Finishers.

Fixers: come as powders or sprays. The setting powder is designed to absorb oil and moisture from your face and the products themselves so that they last longer and don't smudge or melt as you go about your business. A fixer spray sticks to the product without changing it and gives it some hold. Think of them a bit like hairsprays except for your face.

Finishers: are usually translucent powders that help soften the texture of your skin, blur any pores and can give the skin a bit if a glow. A light dusting after you finish your main make up is all that you need. Sometimes they can be used instead of concealer and highlighters if your face is relatively clear of blemishes and already has some femme features.

If we need to build up layers of concealer to hide darker tones on our skin we will need a fixer. This is because the creamy nature of the products means they will smudge around with each layer. We fix each one in place so we can build on top. Of course, less is more. Younger females often get this wrong and look heavily made up. The trick is to use as thin a layer as possible and no thinner. Easier said than done.

Products for Eyebrows

Women spend a lot of time grooming their eyebrows, they shape them and pluck them, and brush them to get nice feminine shapes. We will have quite a bit on eyebrows in Part 2 but to get the best results you need a range of things including: brow pencil, pomade, gel and glue (yes glue).

A pomade is a cream based product that usually comes in a little pot. It helps colour your brows to get an even look or fill in sparse areas. Some are waterproof so that the colour will not run in the rain or when you exercise and perspire. It is best to apply the product with a brush.

A brow pencil is used to give more definition to your brows. Usually this means outlining one side of the brow to give a smoother line but it can also be used to fill in missing hair or shape the end of the brow for a more femme look. Over doing your brows to get a drawn on or tattoo effect is one of the most common tells in makeup so again less is more.

An eyebrow gel is similar to hair gel. It helps to keep your brows styled and under control for a smooth look. Gels can also be used to give some volume to your eyebrows if they look flat or to tame overly bushy ones. If your brows are really bushy you need to trim them back for a femme look.

A brow glue is used to hide some of your eyebrows if you don't want to trim them girl fashion. You can use regular craft glue that easily washes out with water. The idea is you spread glue on the brows and then comb them nice and flat. This will give them a couture look. To hide them let the glue dry and then use concealer to paint over the bits you don't want visible (more in Part 2).

Innovations in the cosmetic industry mean that new products become available all the time. Currently there are various combinations of the above which make the application easier and contribute to different looks.

Eye products

For the eyes there are three main products: Eye shadow, Eye liner, and Mascara. The relative amounts of each and how they are applied can lead to all kinds of different looks.

Eye shadow: is simply a colouring for your eyelids. It is called shadow because it goes into the crease between the eyeball and the brow to give a shadow effect. Apart from colours there are all sorts of different materials to carry the colour including powder, cream, liquid, stick or baked shadow. The difference is the spreading and blending ability. The easiest to use for a beginner is powder. Powder eyeshadow comes in different finishes such as matte, shimmer, and satin. Matte is good for everyday use. Shimmer is good for an extra sparkle for the evening and clubs where the light is subdued. Satin gives your eyes a very smooth look good for bedroom eyes or a sophisticated look.

The shadow itself comes in a palette or as individual pans of product. Typical palettes are duo (2) or quads (4) that give you a set of matching or complementary colours. For that everyday look a palette of nudes or beiges will complement your skin tones. For other occasions choose a palette that complements your eye colour. Normally the palette will come with a little applicator (stick with a foam head or little brush). Use that if you want but it is better to use a proper eye brush.

Eye Liner: is a cosmetic that is applied as a line round the eyes to make them appear larger or more noticeable. The liner can come as pencil or as a liquid. The line can be thicker or thinner or shaped to give a more almond or rounder look or some tilt to the overall eye shape. Getting nice neat lines takes a steady hand and finesse so whether you use liquid or pencil depends on your skill level. Liquid is easier to smudge while you apply but gives nicer sweeps. With a pencil you can pet the line to get the right look. Some people lay down the line with a pencil and then touch it up with liquid. The most common colour is black but different colours can complement your eyes and shadow.

Mascara: is a carbon black or iron oxide mix that darkens your eyelashes. Modern versions include a polymer that coats the lashes and waxes or oils to give the lash extra volume. Big lashes are seen as very feminine and attractive. Females do have longer thicker lashes than males so mascara will help feminize your eyes. They also make your eyes look bigger. The most popular colour is black but you can also use brown if your eyebrows or complexion is lighter or to complement your eye colour. Most products come with an applicator brush which can be shaped to make it easier to get the mascara on the lash without smudging your eyeshadow and also to help give the lash a nice curl.

Lip Products

For lips there are four basic products. Lipstick, Lip gloss, Balm and Lip liner. You can sometimes use a mixture of these because they have different translucencies and fixing abilities.

Lipstick is a high pigment product which gives a lot of colour to your lips. It can come as a glossy, satin, or matte finish. Matte is more every day, satin can be formal or chic but also bedroomy, and glossy is sexier and more sensual making your mouth look moist and kissable. They come as liquid or as the more traditional bullet form. The bullet makes it is easier to apply colour quickly whereas the liquid needs to be painted on. Most makeup artists will paint your lips because it is easier for them than using a bullet. Vice versa a bullet is easier when you apply it yourself. Some lipstick is waterproof or smudge resistant. Use these if you don't want to leave your lip print on glasses or cups when you drink, smudge off your look when you kiss, or don't want to touch up your lips throughout your girl time. Although, all of these things can be super femme.

Gloss is more translucent and helps seal the lips or lipstick. It can make your lips look softer compared to a matte which is more glamourous and satins which are classy. The gloss often comes with a small brush applicator so you can quickly brush or touch up your lips. Because a gloss has little or no colour your lipstick or natural lip colour shows through. Note though that some people just prefer the glossy version of regular lipstick.

A Balm is mostly used to seal the lip surface to retain moisture and keep them from cracking or drying out in hot or cold weather. They come in a variety of shades or tints such as pink, red, peach, or brown so can be used to accent your own lip colour. Some also have different flavours. Whereas the lipstick is full colour and the gloss is transparent the balm is somewhere in between. They come in a bullet form or as a small pot. In the former you can cover your lips in a similar way to lipstick and for the latter can use a finger to rub the Balm into your lips. If your skills are such that lipstick is still a challenge or you are on the go a bit of balm can give you a nice femme look in virtually no time. However, it is often not strong enough in colour to balance full makeup.

Lip liner helps to define your lips. You outline the border between your lip and the rest of the muzzle area and so can define your mouth better. Depending on how it is done this can make your lips look bigger or smaller. You can apply a balm or primer before the lip lining stage. Altogether this makes your lips smoother and creates an outline for you to follow with lipstick. Usually a liner comes as a pencil. Once the lips are outlined it is easier to apply your lippy nice and smoothly. A little touch up with concealer and you can have nice crisp looking lips like those old-style movie actresses or a beauty pageant contestant.

Basic Brushes

Now we have all these products the next challenge is to get them onto your face in a way that makes them look good. We've mentioned some forms of applicators like pencils and bullets but when we are talking about powders and creams, we need brushes and a few other things to be able to work the product and blend them together.

The range and number of makeup brushes is staggering. A make up artist might have 32 or more different brushes. They need that many because they do lots of different styles. If you look online or in a store you will see all sorts of brush sets and a wide range of prices. What is a girl to do! Don't get overwhelmed. You only need a few to make a decent job. Here are the top five most essential brushes:

A face brush: is for applying your foundation. It has a dome shape to pick up product and to allow you to spread it on your face and work it to blend.

An angled brush: is for applying blush and bronzer and to give you some contouring. Smaller ones can also be used for applying eyeliner and touching up detail.

A fan shaped brush: is for applying highlighter to bring out the high parts of your features- normally the nose and brow (or T-bar), tops of cheek, and chin areas (I-bar).

A fluffy powder brush: is for dusting the face to apply finishing powder or bronzer or whatever lightly all over the face.

An eyeshadow blender brush: this again is dome shaped but smaller and a little stiffer than the face brush. It allows you to pick up product from the palette or pan and place it accurately onto the eyelid and then work and blend it along the crease or lid shape.

That's all you need to get started. As you get into this, you will start to appreciate how particular types of brush help you get the look you want. As your skill develops you might want to invest in smaller angled brushes for precise and detail work, or more dense crease brushes for the eyes. We have already mentioned lipstick brushes and eyeliner brushes too. Like painting, it isn't the brush it's how you use it that matters. The more expert you get the more you will want to extend your range. More than one of each type of brush allows you to load up the brushes with different skin tones and colours to help define your look and speed up the application. For example, with a different brush for primer, foundation, and concealer or different colour correctors.

Brushes vary in price quite a bit and it is important to understand what you are paying for. A good brush is an investment, with proper cleaning and storage they can last for years. And, you will have your favourites. You might also want a classy home set and a cheaper (small) set that you can carry about for touch ups when you are out. The brush fibres can be natural hair or synthetic. The quality of the brush fibre affects its ability to pick up, transfer, and deposit the product. Man-made ones usually contain polyester which makes them softer and more absorbent. This means they are better for work with concealers and less prone to damage from cleaning products. A natural fibre brush traps more product and is made of animal hair. Stiffer brushes are better for things like foundation and softer brushes for spreading and blending so always test the bristles before you buy to see if it will meet your needs.

Clean your brushes regularly. The oils from your face and the build-up of residue from your products can make them stiffer and harder to use over time. Also, they are prone to collect bacteria and other nasties which feed off your body oils. Use a mild cleanser to keep them clean and in good condition. A Baby shampoo which is both soft and gentle is ideal.

Accessories and other bits

There are a few other things that might be worth considering as an investment or to help with your look.

Sponges: brushes will get the job done but sometimes you need to accelerate the process. One area where this is true is if you are using creams and don't want to mess up your powder brushes. A shaped (triangular, wedge, or round) sponge can be used for quick application of foundations and concealer to get a preliminary blend and to block out your face. Round ones fit on the contours of your face better but the triangular ones can be used for precision delivery. Powder puffs that come with some products can also be used instead of brushes. You'll see these in compacts or when a girl needs to powder her nose or touch up the chin area.

Eyelash curlers: are a clever little invention that can be used to crimp your upper lid lashes and give them extra curl which opens up your eyes. Use them before you apply mascara so that the lash is more accessible or instead of if you are in a rush or don't want to volumize the lash.

False Eyelashes: men have less lash material than women so if mascara is not working for you or you find it difficult to apply use false lashes. These fit over your own lashes to give more volume and you can get further extension with Mascara. More on this in Part 2.

Tweezers: are essential for fine tuning your eyebrows and picking out the odd wayward hair. Once you know the shape of your brows you can use them to pluck hairs to get a lovely femme shape rather than waxing or shaving. They are also invaluable to extend your reach and allow precision placement of false eyelashes in difficult to reach areas.

Compacts: every girl should have a makeup compact. One side holds extra powder for a touch up and the other contains a mirror. Slip them in your bag so that you can check your makeup easily and adjust as necessary. The mirror also allows you to see difficult places like eye detail and/or lipstick. They also help with applying the product. You will have to learn to use one properly but it is the most femme thing ever to use your compact in public or while you are waiting for someone.

Pencil Pots and Brush Rolls: you have to keep all this stuff somewhere. The products all come with containers so you just need a surface or some draws. But think about getting a pencil pot for your eyeliner, lipliner, and other pencil products. Brushes can also be stored in pots but many girls like a little wallet or a fabric roll that they can slot the brushes into and then tidy them away.

Makeup Bag: there are a wide variety of bags to hold your products ranging from girly girl ones to more sober functional ones with plastic linings in case of a spill. If you have a big range of cosmetics then choose only the ones you are wearing and slip the containers into your makeup bag with a few brushes and a compact or small mirror and carry them in your handbag so you can touch-up on the go. Less is more -essentials only.

Tissues/cotton buds, wipes: you'll also need some things that can be used to mop up excess product and to clean up smudged areas that are too small for a brush. Wipes help to get all that product off your face. Of course, you also need and may already have moisturizers, exfoliation scrubs, and spot creams to generally pamper your skin when you do take your face off.

Makeup Cleanser: usually you can just use soap and water to get product off your face. This is more difficult though if you have waterproof products like mascara which are designed not to run. Soap also dries out your skin, so you will need to moisturise after. A cleansing milk or makeup and/or eye removal cream makes life easier. Cleansers contain small amounts of oil which helps lift the product.

Take off your eye makeup first (this is the hardest) and then move onto the rest of your face. For the eyes gently work remover into the area then use a flat cotton wipe to take it off. For the face spread cleanser onto your hands and then wash your face as normal. Go back with wipes for the reluctant bits. Don't rub too hard otherwise you'll strip the skin and make it sore – gentle is better. Products like Vaseline (petroleum jelly) will remove eye makeup and Swarfega will also work as a general remover. Vaseline, for example, can also be used as lip balm, to smooth down your eyebrows (though not cover them) and as protection from hair dyes. It also contains Aloe Vera which is nice to your skin.

Shopping list

Well, gosh and golly, there is quite a lot of stuff there! Are you sure you want to be a girl? Just, kidding. But seriously, how much is all this going to cost? Well, how long is a piece of string? It depends on your budget and how addicted to making up your face you are. It is estimated that the average female spends in the order of 30-40 dollars/pounds on products per month. If your income is higher you can afford to indulge and splurge on products. If things are tight stick to the essentials.

Here is your shopping list:

*Primer, Foundation**, *Concealer**, *Blush**, *Highlighter, Bronzer**, *Fixer*

Pomade, brow pencil, eyebrow gel, brow glue

Eye shadow **, *Eye Liner* **, *Mascara* **, *Eyelash curlers, False Eyelashes and Fixing gel*

Lipstick **, *Gloss, A Balm, Lip liner* *

Face brush *, *angled brush* *, *fan shaped brush**, *fluffy powder brush* *, *eyeshadow blender brush* **

*Sponge applicators**, Tweezers, *Tissues/cotton buds,*

*Wipes***, *Makeup Cleanser***

Makeup Compact, Pencil Pots and Brush Rolls, Makeup Bag *

If you need to reduce your upfront investment the most essential items are marked with an asterisk. With this minimal set you should be able to get going and then decide what else you want to buy as you get more into it. You'll also be able to try out most of the techniques in this book. You can reduce further if you just go for the eye and lip items with built in applicators (see double asterisk) but that will make it difficult to do any detailed facial feminization work such as contouring. In this case just try the bits of the book you have the stuff for and then buy more as you want to explore.

Another alternative is to look for gift sets. There are some quite nifty makeup kits available in the £/$25 range if you shop around online. Read through the contents and tick off the items on the above list. The plus side is that you can probably get a nice carry case as part of the package. This solves your storage problems and can also be used for travelling. If you femme up when you are on business trips or go away for the weekend that is ideal. The downside is that you get the foundation skin tones, blush, eyeshadow and lipsticks that come with the kit. These may not be the colours you want or need but they will be coordinated. They are okay as starter kit to try out your technique. You can get more matched skin-tones later when you need to refill. Some Crossdressing stores also do boxed makeup kits and refills but these can tend to be more expensive than the above. One reason for this is that they often have darker tones and thicker or specific colour correcting concealers that help with male features like beard outlines. Your choice.

A starter brush set with 5-8 brushes shouldn't cost you more that £/$10. Foundation and concealer sets £/$10-20 and primer £/$10. In fact, most single items should be in the £/$10 or less price category. Things like disposable mascara wands around £/$4 and single lipstick £/$3-5. A chain store or small brand might be £/$5-10 and fashion house name £/$15 and upwards. Eyelash curlers are around £/$7 and a cheap compact £/$5 ranging up to £/$20+ for metal ones with nice decorative detail. Eye shadow palettes are about £/$10.

Shadow palettes come in all sizes, some with a big range of colours. It is more economic to buy smaller sets with shadow you will actually use rather than big ones with extra colours you are never going to use. All these products have a shelf life. Primers, Foundations, and Concealers last about two years. Cream things like eyeshadows, highlighters, and some blush last only about one year. Eyeliners and stuff in pencils can go three years. But liquids, like mascara, only last about six months. Powders tend to last the longest. Once you open the product the clock is ticking.

If you dress regularly or are a 24/7 girl this will not be too much of a problem but if your dressing is occasional you may find you have to buy more product to replace unused items. The affordability is something to think about when you are choosing your look. Every girl knows that you buy cheaper stuff for everyday and expensive stuff for special occasions. Only well-heeled or professional women can afford expensive cosmetics for day-to-day use. That is why girls go crazy when you buy them those combo sets or why they add it to the birthday or wish list.

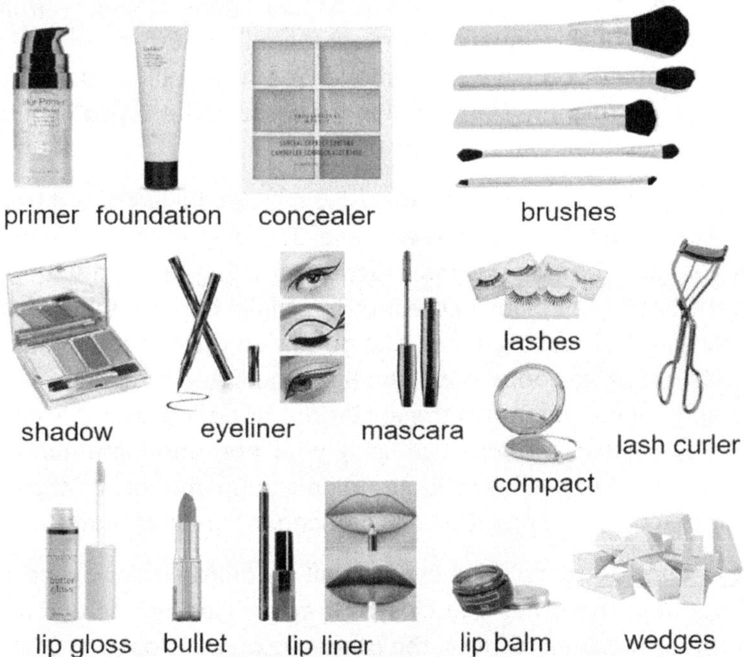

Figure 3 A collection of makeup products and accessories

Basic Skills

Once you get your stuff, you will need to start practicing some skills. You can learn these on the job as you do your make up but you can also build up your technique without wasting makeup products.

<u>*Blending:*</u> is an essential art to move and mix the product on your face. If you don't blend enough your face will have sharper angles and look more male. If you blend too much there will be no contour or definition and the tones will all come out as a muddy mess. What you need is just enough to give rounder softer features but no more. You can practice this with some softer drawing pencils (2B, 5B etc) and some cotton

wool. Draw different patches with lighter and dark shades next to each other on a piece of paper and then practice blending them together with the cotton wool. When you can do that put a bit of product (foundation, concealer, blush) on your face and repeat with your blending brushes.

Dusting: is a finishing type activity that lightly smudges or lifts excess product. For this you use the more fan tail or fluffy brushes. Try that on the samples you have used above. See how it lifts lightens or softens the tones further. The technique is to hold the brush lightly and flick with a very dainty movement of the wrist.

Lining: is the skill you need for using eye and lip liners and to place your shadow precisely in the eye crease. The best exercise for this is to get some colouring books and practice outlining an area with a coloured pencil and then filling in the interior. Make it as neat and as uniform as you can. The real challenge is to do this on the curves of your face. Eyes tend not to be cooperative and lips move. And of course, a mirror flips your image. Sometimes the angles are not good, and it is easier to use the opposite hand. Practice using your non-dominant hand when you colour. To get proficient forget full make up and just do the eyes or lips for practice. This might be all you need in the bedroom.

Eye Control: to do your eyes usually requires that you have one eye open and the other one closed. Practice closing one eye in a relaxed fashion and then focusing the other eye on the closed lid using a mirror. It's harder than you think because your eyeballs usually move together. You might notice that your lid quivers quite a bit which makes it a devil to do detailed work. This is especially true when you are brandishing an eye brush or mascara wand and anticipate a poke in the eye. You will get a reflex (blink) reaction when you touch the lash which you need to learn to control. The more relaxed you are the better. Looking down will also expose more of the lid for treatment which is possible if you use a compact.

Lash control: is another skill which is used when you apply mascara or an eye curler or even putting on your falsies. To get access to the lashes and avoid smudging the rest of your eye makeup you need to push the eye lash out a bit. Do this by keeping your eye half open and then sort of squeezing the muscles around the eyeball. This will flex the upper lid a tiny bit. Again, as soon as you get close to the lid its going to flap to protect your eye so you need to stay relaxed. Sometimes opening your jaw and stretching the muzzle area helps get some stillness. Another approach is to defocus the eye which is the centre of attention or at least to not look at the applicator. Also looking up with the eyeball in question will reduce quivering and help the lash stick out more. Do what you need to do as quickly as possible or in little stages with more control.

Lash Curling: or using an eyelash curler is another essential skill. The device is curved on one side and has a lever or scissor arrangement to open and close a clamp. The concave side goes towards your face and allows the curler to fit your eyelash shape. The trick is to tilt your head back a little and let your eyelash rest between the open clamp (it looks like a guillotine but is blunted or cushioned). Try to keep your eye open. Open the clamp and get it as close to the base of the lash as you can. Operate the levers and the clamp closes onto the lash and bends (or curls) it for a perkier look. Hold the clamp closed for a few seconds. Then open it and move it further out on the lash (about halfway) and repeat. If you want a real curl apply a third time towards the end of the lash. Because male lashes are shorter than female ones two applications per lash is good going. You can also curl false lashes once they are set properly to give them a natural shape and help blend them together with your own lashes. Some mascara will give you extra curl as it dries if this is difficult.

Using a compact (or small mirror): makes it easier to see the angles on your eyes and mouth. Because your eyeballs move together, like they are on a stick, it is easier if you can move the mirror. Hold the mirror with one hand and position it in front of the eye until you can see the area of detail with the non-closed eye and have the best angle for applying the product. This can take a bit of coordination. Remember you are not applying the product to the mirror but to your face. Sounds obvious but trust me, you are going to get confused until you learn the skill. A simple exercise is to just practice touching your face in the right spot using the mirror as a guide.

Common Female looks

In research for this book a simple online search brought up over 1500 different ways to do makeup and style your hair. Everyone has some advice. Where is a girl to start? Here are some common looks that illustrate most of the techniques you will learn in the following pages:

Professional or business look: the emphasis here is on a good foundation to conceal blemishes and eye bags then a hint of colour on the cheeks. Neat but sensible eyes with some contouring and neutral colour on the lips. You will need to master this one if you are a 24/7 girl or are holding down a job ahead of your final transition.

Evening or formal look: this uses a clean foundation and then contouring to provide formal lines of the cheek bones to create a flawless face. Play up your eyes or mouth or both. Maybe use fake lashes or crimp. Gloss up the lips. You will need this one so you can live it up at the nightclub or do social things like a trip to the theatre or a dance.

Couture look: this has a dramatic beauty style with sheer and dewy skin and only a little enhancement on the eyes, cheeks, and lips for a fresh face look. This is popular on the catwalk and makes you appear more like a porcelain doll or a toned-down version of a geisha girl. If you want an English rose look or to understand how contrast can make you look striking this is good practice.

The preppy look: is increasingly popular amongst younger women and is all about glowing skin, long lashes, a hint of blush, and pink lips. The emphasis is on a good or healthy appearance, so you need to have a regular pamper routine, washing and exfoliating your face every night. It also helps if you use primer before your makeup. The effort involved implies that you have leisure time on your hands which indicates status and wealth.

The next day look: has heavy variations on eye liner and natural or almost unstyled hair. Of course, the secret is to style your hair in a way that looks natural or unkempt in a chic kind of way not just leave it untouched. It is called the next day look because it can appear that you didn't take your make up off or redo your hair from the day before. The techniques required for this look will help your overall persona and style whatever it turns out to be.

Girl next door look: this is the archetypical all-American girl style who is cute, fun, and drama free. Typically, she grew up being 'one of the guys' but now has blossomed into an attractive female. Everyone wants to take her home to meet the family. This style is effortlessly gorgeous with makeup suitable for every occasion. It is hard to master. Even females struggle with it. Long term, though, it will give you the most natural and passable look. Mila Kunis, in *that 70s show*, is a good example.

There are of course many other looks including the smoky-eyed rock chick to the trashy or skanky looks where your makeup clashes or dominates to make you look cheap. If you master the above basic looks, it is easy to overdo one aspect or another to get a world-weary appearance. For example, bright red lipstick can look fantastic in a high fashion setting or as formal look but it can also have a French tart quality if you over do the blush and choose a too tight blouse or over short skirt with some fishnet stockings and heels.

How long should it take

A woman can easily spend an hour or more doing full makeup for a formal event. Longer if the detail is complicated. The detailing is the layering required and the time to blend materials like blusher and eyeshadow. Obviously the more practiced you get the faster you can go. Below we give you some average times for varying degrees of detail but keep in mind that if you fuss with your hair too that can sometimes double the time you need.

A simple everyday look with some foundation, a splash of blush, eyeliner, and mascara can take 30 mins or less. A quick eye touch-up and some lip balm might only take 5-10mins. If you give yourself a facial first or clean up the skin, treat spots, or shave it is going to be longer. A crossdresser can easily take 2 hours or more if there is a lot of preparation work to prime the canvas or if they are unskilled and do not go through the process regularly. Artists reckon that it takes about a thousand hours of practice to get good at painting or sketching. If you only do the odd half hour here and there that will take you 20 years. If you do half an hour everyday it will take you about 2 years. Think about it. A teenage girl blossoming into a woman has about three years from 18-21 to perfect her technique. Many, of course, start much earlier than that.

Also, remember that women do this every day before they go to work in the morning and may well do a fuller version in the evening when they go out to socialise. They practice constantly and get proficient. A professional makeup artist that primps fashion models for a living or does special occasion makeup may create a work-of-art in half the time or do make-and-go styles in minutes. They find all sorts of ways to do things quickly, so it is worth watching them work. Youtube and fashion blogs have thousands of hours of videos on how to do different styles of makeup. Try the techniques in this book then look up a video. You may think you are the only one with a given problem but trust me, there will be hours of footage and channels dedicated to solving it. Females love to share secrets.

The takeaway from all this is to make sure you devote enough time to putting on your face. Enjoy being femme and making yourself look good. Play with your hair styles. Your inner girl will be so happy. Learn how to layer up so you have convenient stopping points along the way. And, don't beat yourself up because your early attempts look clumsy. All girls go through these stages. Each time you try you will learn and get a little closer to what you want.

And finally

Okay, so we are almost ready to get on to practical things. First though here are a few more helpful notes. First is getting the right skin tones. Using the wrong tones of foundation, concealer and blush is one of the big rookie mistakes for females, 24/7 girls, and crossdressers alike. Your makeup needs to blend with your own natural skin tone. Females generally have lighter skin tones than males.

When you look online or walk up and down the cosmetic counters, you'll see a bewildering number of choices. It is all very simple though. First you need your basic skin tone which is essentially light, medium or dark. Light skin is usually from Northern Europe where there is plenty of cloud cover all year round. Medium is associated with Southern Europe and North Asia where the skin is more olive coloured. And Dark skins are associated with the Middle East, Africa, and India. In a nutshell your basic skin tone will be darker when you come from a country or have family ties to a country that has a lot of sun and UV radiation. The colour comes from all the melanin used to protect your skin. Each of these three basic tones can have lighter, medium or darker variations giving you a wide range of skin tone products.

The next thing you need to consider is your skin undertone. The undertone comes from how your skin shows things like blood vessels and veins. In other words, how translucent or reflective it is. Basically, your undertone can be warm, neutral or cool. Cool is more pink, yellow-green and bluish. Warm is yellow-orange, reddish, or peachy. Neutral is more olive, greenish-gray, or a mix of warm and cool (that healthy caramel colour). Your complexion is not just about skin and undertones though, it also includes how dry your skin is, the degree of oil, or whether it has a glow.

When you look for the right product keep your skin tone, undertone, and complexion in mind. Look at your skin in natural light and then choose the basic tone. Check out the colour of your veins and determine if they are bluer (cooler) or greener (warmer). See if gold (warm) or silver (cooler) jewellery contrasts with your skin better. How much of an overall gray tone is there? Choose the skin tones that match your basic and undertones. You will also need products one shade lighter and two darker to allow for highlighting and contouring. You can get an idea for this by swatching. That is, laying some of the product on your skin with others and seeing which work best. That is why it is a good idea to go to a store to buy. At least initially until you know what you need.

Another thing to note is that a face primer isn't just for those with oily skin. Many products now have antiaging properties that help support, tighten, or keep the skin healthy. A primer is often a good idea just because it forms a barrier between your skin and other products. This can help improve your overall complexion and with makeup removal. Sometimes they can also have UV screens as well which apart from protecting the skin will help prevent your skin tone changing under your makeup. The former is important because if your skin tans and you have bought one kind of tone that can ruin your look. That is why some women seem to have mismatched makeup when they are on holiday.

Another tip is not to remove your makeup with baby wipes or other types of wet tissues. You may already have these around the house and will find that they are cheaper than makeup wipes. A good baby wipe will remove makeup – well most of it. But here's the thing. You still need to follow up with makeup cleanser. Makeup wipes are built to dissolve product and remove more of it. Micellar water also does a good job. If you leave traces of makeup, then this can block pores and lead to spots and other skin breakouts. And, you need to do a thorough job because leaving a hint of shadow, mascara, or foundation will give your secret life away.

And, last, don't steal your makeup. No, really. What we mean by this is sneaking into your partner's or housemate's boudoir and using her stuff. First up, it is not necessarily going to match your skin tone, complexion, or eyes. Second, she will notice. If you use the brushes differently, load them up with different colours, and do not clean them properly she's going to get suspicious. Especially if you use her special occasion products. And, hey, this stuff is expensive. She's going to know how long it is supposed to last. You're also likely to smudge applicators, bottles, and other containers especially if you are clumsy or ham-fisted putting it on or getting it off. And, unless you have an extraordinary eye for detail, you are not going to put it all back in the right places. Yes, she may lend you stuff or use her own products if you are playing together but that is her choice. The decent thing to do is buy your own stuff. Enough, said.

Part 2
Putting on your Face

"Beneath the makeup and behind the smile I am just a girl who wishes for the world."

—Marilyn Monroe

"Beauty, to me, is about being comfortable in your own skin. That, or a kick-ass red lipstick."

—Gwyneth Paltrow

Chapter 4 Priming the canvas

In this part we will look at how to create a more feminine looking face. Of the four-stage method outlined in chapter one we will cover the first three stages. The final stage of hair styling and accessories is covered in Part 3. Skip there now if you are happy with your makeup choices or don't need any help disguising your male features.

The first thing we look at in this chapter is how to prime your face and get it ready for more detailed work on the eyes and lips later. The key to success is to have some basic understanding of colour theory or how different colours work and combine to create different effects. Don't worry we aren't going to overload you with nerd stuff. But this really helps. You will then be able to choose the right colour concealers to hide male facial hair such as beard growth and eyebrows effectively as well as make your eyes and lips 'pop' with vitality.

The next chapter covers basic contouring. We will look at the shape of your face and how to make it appear more girl-like. There are two parts to this. First is the angularity of the perimeter of your face and the way it hugs the hair and jaw line. We look at how to make this softer and rounder. The second part is the surface of your face or how it undulates and curves to make features. For this we will introduce the idea of facial planes and show how they can be used with different makeup tones to give you more feminine cheeks, reduce or disguise the brow ridge and give you a more petite looking nose.

The third and fourth topics are eyes and lips. In those chapters we will show you how to apply your shadow and give yourself eye wings so that your eyes look more almond and have that typical female slant. We'll also show you a simple tip or two to deal with the dreaded hooded eye problem. Then we will look at lips and how to make your mouth appear smaller and more femme as well as giving you the appearance of more plump. Of course, none of these techniques actually change your underlying features but we can alter how people see or perceive your face. That's pretty cool all by itself.

How to prime

We covered primer in the last chapter. If you recall it helps to even out your skin tone and blur any blemishes. The right formulation will help with anti-aging and moisturise your skin to give a natural healthy glow. If your complexion is very clear and you don't have much male hair growth on your face you may be able to just wear primer for an everyday look. If you mix primer with foundation rather than as separate layers it can give you a dewy skin look.

Anyways, first things first. The major reason to use primer is to make your skin extra smooth so that all the other products will go on more easily. Most primers will help with overall redness or other blotchy things making it easier for concealers and foundation to be more effective. Overall, this means that you can use less product and layers to get a clean look. Nothing worse than having to cake on the concealer so that your finished face appears makeup heavy.

Before you start applying the primer make sure you have washed, exfoliated, treated any spots, and shaved nice and closely. Use a gentle astringent after you shave to close up the pores. Then apply your favourite moisturiser. Once you are all clean and ready apply the primer as follows. Take a small amount (about the size of a fingernail) and use your fingertips to spread and blend it all over your face making sure you get good coverage. Go all the way to the side of the cheekbones and under your eye sockets, forehead, and out to the side of the jaw line. Add a bit more under your chin and down over your natural beard line. You get the idea.

Colour-Correcting

The next thing we do is to apply concealer over major blemishes, beard, and brow area. Before you do that it is worth taking a few moments to understand the basics of colour theory. People get confused about all this and so tend to just use a standard concealer. Do that and you're missing out on one of the best techniques to get a nice femme look and use the minimum amount of product. That is going to help you appear more passable and save you money. It's a win-win, so stick with it.

The principle is easy. Remember painting in school when you had to mix colours up and didn't have the right one? For example, a brown when you only had the colours red, blue or yellow. If you wanted a more purple brown then you added more blue. For a lighter brown you added more yellow. And for a greyer brown more red. That is what colour theory is about. It tells you how to mix colours and what colours work best with one another. For example, we mix primary colours (red, blue, yellow) to get secondary colours (green, orange, and purple) and other colours by mixing primary and secondary colours. A primary colour is one that cannot be made from other colours.

Now, just before you jump in and say that the primary colours are Red, Green and Blue. It depends on the colour system you are using. When we mix products like paint or concealers or eye shadow, we are using the subtractive system. When scientists talk about light, they use the additive system. Here's why. When light hits an object some of it is absorbed and the rest is reflected. So mixing paints or product is like deciding which colours you don't want to reflect (that is subtraction). But when we see an object our eyes combine the reflected light using the Red, Green, and Blue recognising cells in the back of our eyes (that is adding). As long as you understand whether something is reflecting or observing it is easy to remember which primaries apply.

Okay, can you begin to see where we are going with this? When you buy cosmetics like lipstick and eye shadow the product is already mixed to give the colour you want. You just buy the right shade. But to conceal something or correct its colour we need to think about what we need to mix with it to change what we see. And, ideally, what we want to see is a nice skin tone. Let's put that a different way. What colour is your 5 O clock shadow? Is it a bit blue, grey, has a hint of green or maybe a mixture? Or perhaps you have some red pimple marks. How can we make them appear more skin like and magically disappear from your face? What colour mix should we use to absorb (or subtract) the colour you don't want to see?

To understand which colours to use for this little piece of magic we need a colour wheel. The wheel is easy to construct if you remember that little rhyme about colours of the rainbow. Richard Of York Gave Battle In Vain (or Red, Orange, Yellow, Green, Blue, Indigo, Violet). If we combine Indigo and Violet as just shades of Purple there are just six colours. Notice that the primaries are then all separated by secondary colours. If you combine Red and Yellow, you get Orange; Yellow and Blue gives Green; Blue and Red gives Purple. Arrange them in a circle and you have your colour wheel.

Now, every colour on the colour wheel has an opposite or complementary colour. For each of the secondary colours the complementary colour is the primary that wasn't used to make it. Orange is made from Red and Yellow, so its complementary colour is Blue. The complementary for Green is Red. And for Purple it is Yellow. Notice that the complementary colour is almost directly opposite the colour you have on the colour wheel. Knowing this allows you to quickly choose a good colour to make your starting colour stand out or to choose a colour to hide or subdue another colour. That's why cosmetic companies give you those little swatch cards.

When we put a colour and its complement next to each other the contrast between them appears increased. The reason for this is that colour from the opposite side of the colour wheel are either warm (Red, Orange, Yellow) or cool (Green, Blue, Purple) and so we are contrasting a warm and cool colour. That's what we call 'pop'. Everything somehow looks more vital and jazzy. It's a trick of how we perceive colours with our eye. We will be using all this later to make your eyes have more twinkle but right now let's make your beard area disappear. When we mix warm and cool colours, we put all the primary colours back together. If you absorb all the colour nothing is reflected (which is black). But this is quite hard to do. Most often what we see is a more subdued or in between colour which is referred to as neutral. This can be used to tone things down a bit. And, more importantly for feminization purposes it creates a muddy colour.

Did you get that? A mixture of a warm and cool colour will tend to produce a brown or tanned skin colour. For example: Yellow and Purple (lighter tone); Red and Green (mid-tone), Blue and Orange (darker tone). So, for the best outcome, the colour of the concealer needs to be matched with the colour you want to cover up. If your skin looks tired or grey use pink shades. For hyperpigmentation use yellow, for dark bluey-purple under eye circles use peach or orange, for dull or sallow (yellowy) skin use lavender, and for redness use green. Consider that for a moment. If your beard shadow has a green tinge you need a bit of red in your concealer. If you have a bit of blue-green, then some orange in the concealer will muddy things up. Get the idea?

Beard concealment

Armed with our knowledge of colour theory it is straightforward to hide your beard. Take a look at the shade of skin in your chin area. Even though you have just shaved, the hair underneath the skin will give it a certain shade. The colour will vary depending on how much hair you have, how much growth a day you get, the colour of your hair, the colour of your skin, and your skin undertones. Choose the right colour concealer using the above list for the shade of your skin. If it already looks a good skin tone or you can not differentiate it from the rest of your face, lucky you!

Now apply the concealer to the area using a sponge or brush. A sponge is faster. Get a nice thin layer and even coverage. Then let it dry a little and apply a finishing powder or fixer to seal it all in. For the best effect you want to fade (or blend) the concealer into the rest of your face at each stage. This will avoid creating a tell-tale outline or bump of material that could show through the rest of your make up. Start by filling the general area with a thin layer of the concealer and then blend out to create a soft edge. Take a look and see how visible the area is or how masked it appears. If you need to, add more layers until the beard shadow has just about disappeared. It is balance between the number of layers and the amount of product on your face. And, don't forget that after this we are going to add foundation over the top which adds another layer.

Figure 4 illustrates the process. If you have only a light growth you might be able to get away with the partial coverage rather than the fuller one. Less is always more when it comes to concealer. Always seal the product with fixer between each layer otherwise the layers will just smush together and all you will be doing is pushing increasing amounts of product around on your face without building up the coverage. Another factor to consider is your overall skin tone. The more concealer you add the darker the tone will become so try and use less layers if you have lighter skin and use more if your skin is darker. For example, if you use an orange-based concealer you will start to look more Donald Trump. Use lighter shades of the orange if this is a significant problem or use more pinkish tones if your beard has a more gray-blue look.

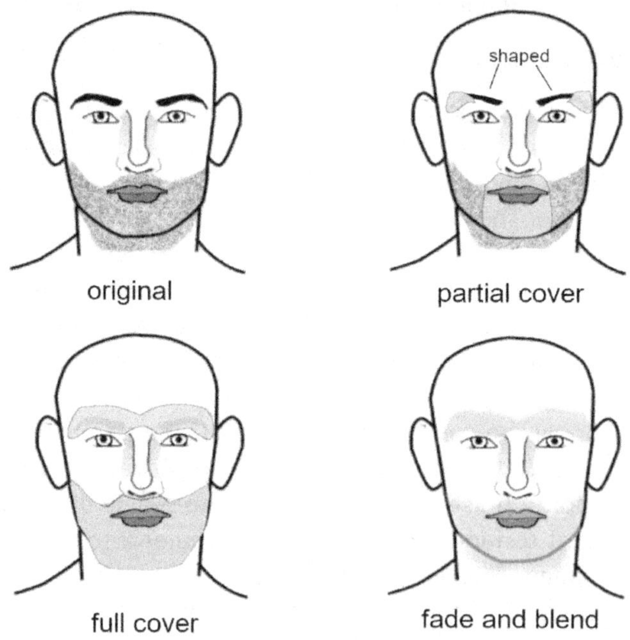

Figure 4 Concealing the brows and beard

Prepping the brows

The next step is to get your eyebrows ready. First, we prepare the brows and then apply concealer to make them disappear. Figure 4 shows the basic areas to consider. The key thing you need to decide is whether you want to style your own brows or are going to cover them over and re-position. If you do the latter, you can keep man brows when you are not dressed. This sounds ideal but you may look false when you do dress because you will be effectively recreating them by drawing or painting them on like a kind of temporary tattoo. It is a personal choice but some real hair on the brows can look very sensual and very femme when shaped correctly. Minimal interference is the best approach to get the look you want. We'll cover all the techniques. So it is up to you.

If your brows are really bushy you will have to trim them down a bit. You can flatten them with concealer and so forth but generally not enough to hide them away. Use a grooming tool like an eye brow or beard trimmer and shave them down so you still have hair but it fits closer to the skin. The next thing is shape. By far the simplest thing to do is to actually trim your brows into a girl shape. That is, leaving them wide at the nose and tapered as you move out to the side. This is obviously desirable if you are a 24/7 girl. If your feminization is a secret that will not be a realistic option. But it does make your look more passable by a mile.

A happy medium is to shape them a little. Contour them up to the edge of the eye socket before it turns downwards and onto the side of your face then shave (wax or cream) everything else off. The part where they move from the front to the side of your face is where male and female brows differ most. Female ones arch over and away from the socket. Male ones hug the side of the socket. If you get rid of the side hair your brows will look shorter and sit more or less over the eyes. That is still a passable male brow. Then, when you dress you can apply concealer and make up to the outer portion to create a girl shape. This way you get real hair on the inner parts and a pencilled in look on the outside. Many female brows have this appearance. The chapter on eyes shows you how to style them so the key thing now is to get them prepped and ready.

Once the brows are prepped take an eyebrow brush and some craft glue that is easy to remove with soap and water. A typical glue stick from a local stationary shop is fine. Take the brush and comb all the eyebrow hairs nice and flat so they run in the same direction (up and over your eye towards the side). Next apply the glue and slick all the hairs flat to your face. Combing them first makes this step easier. Allow the glue to set a little and then apply fixing powder to dry up any further sticky spots. Next choose the right colour correcting concealer for your brow hair-glue mix and apply a good layer over the whole of the eyebrows and blend it in all along the brow ridge including the side of the eye sockets and just under the ridge. Don't get it on your eye lids though – we don't want to get too thick there for when we apply eye shadow etc. Plus, it will make your eyelids stiffer and more difficult to blink or open your eyes.

If you want to retain a more natural eyebrow look then apply a variation of this technique. Don't glue everything down. Just the outside and/or under edges of the brows where you want to continue with girl brows and then apply the concealer to the side of the socket and blend it into the rest of the brow ridge. Go around the socket to cover any of the places that you have shaved off just for good measure.

Fix the concealer in the same way you did for the beard area and build up layers if you need to. However, in this case we are going to reconstruct girl brows over the top, so it doesn't matter if some of the colour shows through. No one will be able to see it when we are done. Thicker concealer can also act as a filler so if you blend appropriately on the top of the brow line and just under where the nose starts you can lessen the brow ridge a little and fade it in more to the forehead so that it looks more female.

Foundation

Okay, nearly there. The next step is to apply your foundation. This will provide a uniform smooth skin-tone all over your face and cover the areas you have been working on with concealer. There are a few do's and don'ts here which will avoid moving the concealer and spoiling what you have achieved so far.

The key is not to work the areas of concealer too much. Lightly dab on the foundation in these areas using a brush or a sponge just to get a thin film of coverage. For the rest of the face work the product around so that you get a nice even and smooth coverage all over your face. Once you are done if there are any blemishes still showing through touch up with more concealer and blend it all in for that flawless look. Take a look at Chapter three if you are not familiar with makeup brushes.

If you are using a powder foundation put a small amount of product on your face and work it in. Don't focus on just one area build up the coverage all over your face at the same time. This way you will use the minimum amount of material and avoid chasing around your face trying to match up the depth and coverage. Takes a bit of practice to do it quickly. Always keep your eye on the emerging picture of your whole face rather than the area you are working on at that moment.

If you prefer a cream foundation you can speed things up by using the dot and dab method. Take small amounts of product and put a dab on each of the major planes of the face (see figure 2, chapter 2). Now quickly work the product in using a brush or sponge and blend the patches together– again taking care not to get too involved with the areas with concealer underneath. Just touch them over to get coverage. With a little practice you will soon learn how much product you need in a dab to get a quick and even application.

Eye circles and minor blemishes

The next area to consider is under the eyes where you might have some discolouration or saggy skin that make hollows or eye bags. There are all sorts of ways to alleviate eyes bags using various creams and lotions which we won't go into. For example, putting used tea-bags on your eyes or cucumber as part of a pamper routine or facial. But for a quick fix you can use concealer.

Use the correct colour to hide the discoloration and build up some of the product if you have eye hollows or wrinkles to hide them a bit (it won't take them away completely). If the hollows are deep you might want to invest in some filler products. And apply all this before your primer and foundation. There are a range of revitalising products on the market. Usually they take the form a serum which is absorbed by the skin and gives it more plump. They can be bought in most cosmetic stores or pharmacies that carry beauty products and must be applied regularly (daily) to get any value so make it part of a pamper routine. These are different to the dermal fillers which last longer and where a cosmetic surgeon will inject the filler into your face.

Usually people apply foundation first and then touch-up patches that show through. This is a good idea as it often uses less product and gives you thinner layering overall. Plus, you don't have to be that careful applying the foundation and moving the concealer underneath. You must do the chin/beard area and the brow line before using foundation though because they are so much bigger. Minor blemishes and under eyes can be done after foundation. That is really your last step to set the canvas for your more detailed work. Have a quick check in the mirror and use spots of concealer and blend in for anything minor flaws still showing through. Hopefully you now have a nice even base skin-tone all over your face.

Putting it all together

Here is a helpful little summary of the process so far, we will include these in each chapter so you can see the whole process at one go, and build in the various techniques:

Step 1: wash shave, exfoliate, close-up pores and moisturise your face. Trim your eyebrows for the look you want. Prime your face.

Step 2: choose a colour correcting concealer to mask the beard area and apply. Fade the edges out into the rest of the face and fix for each layer. [Two or three layers should be plenty but stop when you have enough coverage]

Step 3*:* comb your eyebrows flat, glue in place, fix the glue with powder, choose the right correcting concealer and then cover the brow ridge working around any eyebrow you are keeping exposed. Add layers as necessary. Work the bossing just above the nose to flatten the contour a little.

Step 4*:* apply your base skin tone foundation. Be gentle on areas of concealer and blend all over to get a nice smooth finish. [try the dot/dab method if you are using cream-based product].

Step 5*:* add appropriate concealer to cover any under-eye circles and other blemishes still visible. Blend into the foundation.

Remember that a sponge is often quicker than a brush for getting a lot of concealer onto your face. Brushes though will give you a smoother finish so use a mixture to load an area and then blend. Also, if you are using different correctors load them up using different brushes and/or sponges so that you don't mix up material. If you have limited brushes wash them out and dry after you complete a step.

Top Tip: while you are layering do Step 2 and Step 3 together. While the beard area sets properly do the brow and vice-versa. This will save you time.

In fact, you can streamline the whole process depending on how femme your features are or how often you are doing makeup. For example, if you are a 24/7 girl or regular dresser then it makes sense to contour your eyebrows to make them more female. In that case you can miss out most of step 3. And if you are happy with your brow bossing forget it completely. Likewise, you can miss out Step 2 if your beard area is not that visible or if you have the hair permanently reduced or eliminated using laser treatments or electrolysis. Temporary techniques like waxing, threading or depilatory creams can last longer than shaving especially if the hair is softer so you may get several makeup sessions in without the need for concealer. And, guess what. If you only have steps 1, 4, and 5 in your process you're a regular girl anyway.

And finally

We have talked about concealer quite a bit in this chapter and we are not done with it just yet. Here are a few more notes that could be useful.

You might be thinking, why bother with applying all these layers and that colour correcting nonsense. Just buy a thicker more opaque concealer and do it all once. That is an option and might be your only option if you have difficult to hide features like acne scars or deeper hair colour. However, thinner and fewer layers are better because we want to allow your face to move without cracking or creasing the product on your face. If it is too thick you will look like an expressionless wax work. Thinner concealer means layering and colour correction.

Often concealer is lighter than your base skin tone. When you apply it, it can seem a little out there on your face but stick with it. When you add the layer of foundation it will even up quite nicely and of course the lighter coat helps the base skin tone to show up better. Don't apply the foundation too thinly though otherwise it will peep through. Then you'll look a little pale like a china doll.

The actual concealer product comes in different types including liquid, stick, or cream forms. The liquid gives thinner layers but is difficult to get the cover up. And you don't need to seal after each one, just let it dry. In fact, if you do fix liquid concealers then the fixer will gather up and crease to leave an impression when you smile or move you face muscles. A stick is easier to apply for thick coverage and a cream is easier to blend. Most people use cream like formulations. A concealer is made from oils and corn starch among other things so can be quite greasy to the touch. That's why with a cream it is easier to apply a layer and fix it. Otherwise all the layers become one grease paint mess and you'll keep unearthing your blemishes or 5 O'clock shadow as you work the product. So layering is the thing. By the way you can get vegan concealers if that is important to you.

It can take a bit of practice to get the right balance of concealer opacity and thickness for the number of layers and the look you want. If you have difficult areas, then use a more opaque concealer. And, if the regular cosmetic brands don't work for you then look at professional and theatrical concealers. These are designed for camera work like TV presenting, film, and special effects make up. They will blitz any acne problem and can even cover up tattoos. A professional six-colour concealer circle which includes the shades we discussed above can cost up to £/$30 (e.g. Kryolan). Camouflage Crème comes in one colour pans for about £/$5 which you can match to your skin tone. If you buy your makeup from a crossdressing store, more than likely, you will get these thicker concealers in the kit. But always worth asking.

Chapter 5 Basic Contouring and Highlighting

The next step in feminizing your face is contouring. Basically, this means to add lighter and darker shades to your foundation base to create the illusion of soft rounded curves and to pick out more angular features for effect. In addition to your bone structure the outline of your face can make you look softer or more angular. Things like the width of your cheekbones, the shape of the forehead and the squareness of your jaw all add angles to the perimeter of your face. We will look at the common face types and then how to create the most common female shape.

After that, the theme shifts to the planes of the face. This simplified model of your actual contours is used by artists (including makeup artists) to understand how light is reflected off your face. The angle of any light falling on your face casts shadows, so some areas appear darker or lighter than others. This is the concept of value. If an artist copied the right values onto a flat sheet of paper the face drawn would look very realistic. If we play with the value (or light and dark) on your face we can make it look different. We'll show you how to use this trick to create the illusion that your face is a different shape to the way it is.

Next, we will consider how blushers and highlighters are used to create a more feminine look in the centre of the face. This uses a similar principle to value except that different colours of your skin tone are used to create contrast and a healthy-looking glow. It allows us to create feminine cheek bones (or apples) and to make the nose and brow appear smaller or narrower. To appreciate what is going on here, check out that notorious music video -*addicted to love,* by Robert Palmer. The backing group are all women. Their hair is pinned back out of the way and they all have identical makeup, shadow, and lippy. The foundation is a bit pale for the camera but notice how the face shape and body frame influences how feminine each one looks.

Face Types

The literature has a range of different face types and the numbers vary from 4 or 5 basic types to over ten. Below we consider nine face types that are based on angularity versus softness. Nine might seem like a lot to remember but once you get the idea you will see that there is a simple pattern. They cover all the other face types that people talk about. And, anyhow, unless you are planning a career as a makeup artist you only need to know one, your own.

The first three shapes are all based on whether the sides of your forehead, cheeks, and jaw are more or less on the same vertical. This gives you a blocky sort of look which is seen as more male. A quick test for these shapes is to place a ruler or the spine of a good-sized book flat against the side of your face. If it does not or is difficult to rock back and forward with the pivot point around the side of your cheekbone you are probably one of these shapes.

<u>Square:</u> the square is the most obvious and for this look the width of your face (from ear to ear) is roughly the same as the length (from hairline to chin). If you cut this shape up into a grid with two horizontal and vertical lines to find nine areas or zones, the pupils of the eyes and the corners of the mouth (when relaxed) will be at the interior grid points. That's the rule of thirds (see chapter 2).

<u>Rectangle:</u> this shape is like a square except that the length of your face is longer than the width. When you overlay the face with a grid the thirds in the vertical direction are longer than in the horizontal direction. For example, your nose may appear bigger (longer and thinner). You can also have this shape if the vertical thirds don't match exactly. As in a shorter forehead, or a smaller chin and mouth, or a smaller nose and bigger chin etc. Because it may seem that some of your

features are long compared to other people, a rectangle is sometimes called a long face.

Oblong: the oblong is like a rectangle except that the corners of the rectangle are rounder. So, your face might taper slightly at the top of the hairline. Because of the sharp angles in the corners of these shapes they are typical male shapes but the oblong is a little more female because it allows for a softer jaw-line. When we explore how to manage face types in later chapters, we will assume that you have made a rectangle or long face more oblong using the techniques in the rest of this chapter.

The next three shapes are all typified by softness. To qualify for one of these shapes the ruler or book has to move when you test it against the side of your face. This implies that your face is widest from cheek to cheek and then rounds in towards the top and the bottom. Because of the soft features they are all usually associated with female faces. Although a chubby male can be round, and some male models have a heart shape.

Round: in this shape your face is basically a circle. Again, like the square, the length of your face from hairline to chin is about the same size as the width of your face from cheek to cheek. This length is the diameter of the circle. It is a typical baby face (especially if you are a little chubby). In a baby's face all the features (the eyes, nose, and mouth) are all in the bottom half of the circle. In an adult you might find you have some features like this but normally you can place a square inside the circle in a way that the corners just touch the outline and divide the face up using the rule of thirds.

Oval: the oval is a stretched circle. Sometimes it is more egg-shaped with the circle pulled down at the bottom into a longer shape to form a narrower softer chin. A more extreme version is called a teardrop. This means that the forehead from hairline to cheek is more circular and the bottom more tapered. Normally you can still draw a smaller square/rectangle inside the oval and apply the rule of thirds to get all the facial features. A teardrop version with a squared top is often called a shield.

Heart: in this shape the oval is tapered further with the chin even more pointed. The centre hair line usually forms a widows' peak or is slightly extended down towards the nose in a V-shape. This makes the forehead down to the brow line look more cartoid with the chin forming the point of the heart. The result can be a more defined but smaller jaw and chin. Although many men have the classic M-shape hairline a small number do have the more feminine widows' peak.

The next three face types are all distinguished by more acute angles. Whereas the first three types have perpendicular angles and the second three types have very open angles (or arcs), the following all have sharper angles which are more noticeable as facial features.

Triangle: in this shape the widest part of your face is the distance across the jaw which then narrows as we move up the face with the cheeks narrower before coming to a point just past the hair line. The forehead still has a little width but is narrow compared to the bottom of the face. An inverted triangle does the opposite with the forehead wider than the jaw. The second form is a more female face while the first form is more typical of a male face like a night club bouncer or a boxer. Both males and females can have either type of triangle. The more rounded version is sometimes called a pear shape. And the inverted form is close to a heart shape. Note that some references in the literature flip the names of inverted or non-inverted triangle.

Diamond: this face type is two triangles in which the cheeks (or sometimes the temples) are the widest part and the upper and lower face both narrow towards the hairline and chin. A softer form can also look a little heart shaped. Again, both males and female can have this look but the cheek bones are normally very prominent. A diamond is also called a kite when the upper triangle part is shorter (less vertical) than the lower triangle making the tapered jaw look quite angular. These two features can give it a 'foxy' look especially if the upper part of the diamond is more rounded or heart-like.

Heptagonal: this face type is the most complicated to understand. It is like a diamond with the cheekbones being the widest part of the face. The upper face then tapers in towards the temple but then takes on a more acute angle up to the centre of the hairline. In the lower face the triangle widens to form a larger chin area. If you count, this gives seven angles altogether – two at the cheeks, three more in the upper part of the face, and another two in the lower half. Hence the name heptagonal – *hepta* meaning seven, *gon* meaning corner or angle in Greek.

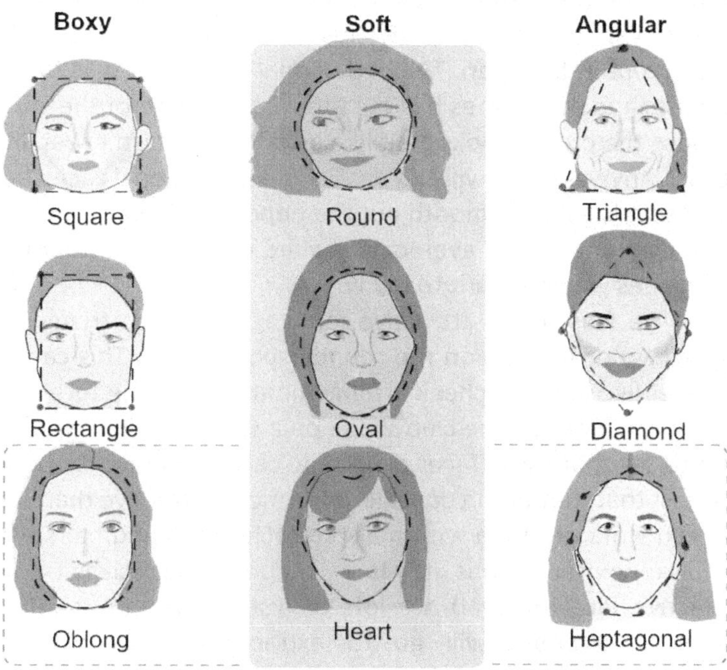

Figure 5 Major Face types

All the above is summarised by Figure 5 with a little rudimentary sketch of a typical face for each type. To make it easy to remember the most female-like faces are highlighted by the shaded area. If we co-opt the oblong as a long female face and note that the heptagonal face can be rounded out quite easily, over half of the types have female qualities. Another distinction is that all the female faces have softer angles this is shown by the dots on the corners of the other faces. If you don't want to apply contouring techniques and go with your natural face type then there are lots of possibilities and we will look at ways of using hair styles to flatter your face in Part 3.

The most common face type for females is the oval and its variations. The next most common face is the heart shape. A diamond shape is the rarest shape which is why it is so memorable and striking. The 'evil' female character in many cartoons or animations have a diamond shape. Think Angelina Jolie in *Maleficent,* the character Cruella De Vil in *101 dalmatians (*squarish diamond*),* or the evil queen in *Snow white (*more heart shaped diamond*).* After diamond, the square is the next rarest female face. Triangles, rectangles, and oblongs are somewhere in between. The heptagonal type is hard to find in female face lists and sometimes has the alternative name of the vampire face because the outline looks a bit like a coffin and it isn't seen in a mirror. Get it? Anyways, we will not talk about heptagonal faces any further because it is easy to smooth out the upper and lower angles to make it more diamond like or even oval shaped using the contouring and hair techniques we are about to study.

The least most attractive female face is the triangle (with the wider jaw) or its relation the rounder pear shape. This can give you a hamster like jaw and cheek arrangement. And, if the forehead is small then it can look like the club shape on a set of playing cards. Now, that isn't to say that these faces cannot be cute and endearing in their own way just that they aren't considered as more attractive than other looks. We can work on them with makeup techniques and hairstyle so don't be disappointed if this it you – keep reading. Likewise, the most attractive face (or oval) has lots of distinction and variations in the literature. Women will go to extraordinary lengths to get an approximation to the oval shape because the beauty industry says this is the ideal type. We will examine all the makeup tricks they use below.

Planes of the Face

The face projects out from the front of your head. The way it curves from the sides of your face to the bridge of the nose are referred to as the contours of your face and are defined by the underlying bones, muscle, and fat. We only ever see the reflected light from an object to make sense of it so the contours can be understood as describing how your face reflects light. This is well understood by artists be it for figure drawing, cartoons, or makeup. We can exploit this fact to trick the eye by applying different tones of makeup to give the impression that light is being reflected differently. This will fool the observer into thinking your face has a different structure. To be successful we need to understand the planes of the face.

The basic and secondary planes of a typical face are the same whether you are male or female and fit inside the perimeter of your actual face shape. For easy reference we have included the planes in the following diagram. An artist creates the contour of the face on a 2D canvas by varying the tones according to these planes and the angle of the light falling on the face. Generally, a darker plane next to a lighter plane will give the idea of depth or curve. Artists call the different shades values. That is easy to understand when you are using just black, grey, and white. All colours have tints (lighter shades) or tones (darker shades) which are different to shadows which are caused by the blocking of light. In practice we will be using colours (or your skin tones). We have your base foundation, the slightly darker shade, and then the shade darker than that. Plus, of course, a lighter shade for picking out detail (or highlights). That is why you need three extra shades of your base foundation. We will use makeup for the tints and tones and leave things like hair length and style to create flattering shadows.

To be successful with this technique you need to master three basic ways the planes are shaded (or coloured) when they share a boundary. A *hard edge* occurs when a tone changes abruptly between two planes. A *softer edge* occurs when the two tones are blended across the boundary line. And a *lost edge* occurs when the blending is so subtle that you barely notice the transition at all. The art to realistic portrait drawing or painting is to copy these subtle changes. In makeup artistry we can make your features look more angular or softer by the way that we blend the foundation tones cross the edges of the planes. And, if we are clever, we can use tints and tones to alter where the planes seem to connect and change the shape of your face.

Finding your Girl face

The first step is to make the perimeter of your face more feminine. This means that we need to cut off the angles and approximate a rounded oval in some way. Why oval? Because it is the most popular female face shape and has the widest possible choices for makeup and styling. It is also the shape that the beauty and cosmetic industry targets. However, just softening your face type a little with the methods below will make you more feminine no matter what your face type. If you already have an oval or even one of the ones in the centre column of Figure 5 you can skip this step. Though you might want to read on to get the perfect girl face.

The basic idea is to take your face type and draw the largest oval shape you can get without going outside the perimeter. This can be a little trickier than it sounds because you cannot usually see what you are measuring. And, even if you can, there are some subtleties between one face type and another which are influenced by your own expectations. You will round out the angles or make them more acute to see what you want to see. Figure 6 illustrates the idea for the most difficult (angular or boxy) face types. Once you understand the principles you can adapt the methods for the more femme faces like the oblong or even the heart shape if the jaw is too prominent.

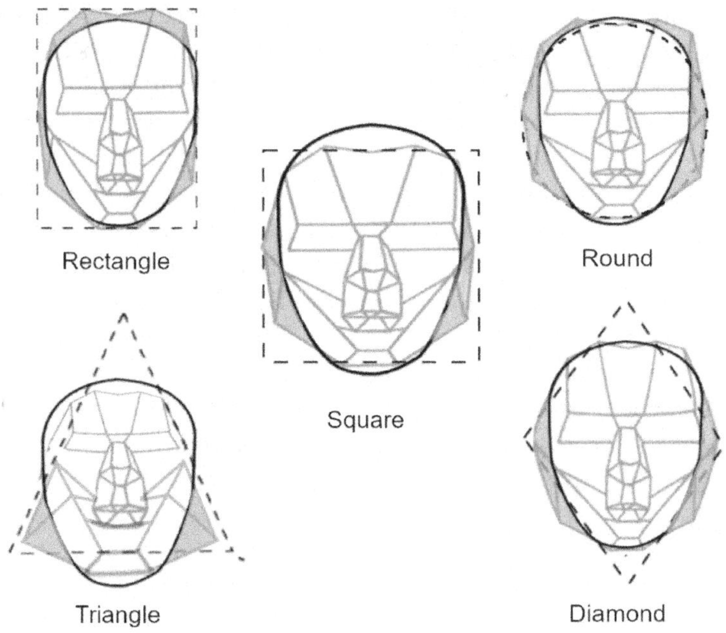

Figure 6 Contouring for face shape

To get an objective view of your face take a lipstick or eyeliner pencil and then trace round the outside of your face as you look at yourself straight on in a mirror. Draw a line from the hair line down to the chin on one side and then around and back up the other side on the mirror. Just follow the angles without rounding out any lines where there is no need to. If you have longer hair. Pull it back and pin it, so you can see the outline of the face. Alternatively, to avoid messing up your mirror, take that virtual makeover pic. Put a piece of thin paper over the top and mark out the face shape with a pencil or pen. You should end up close to one of the shapes in Figure 5.

The next step is to make your face more femme. Draw the largest oval you can make by sticking mostly inside the boundary lines of your sketch. Try to get as close to as many corners as you can while still making a smooth line for the oval shape. You might find that the oval stretches into a tear drop or becomes more rounded, egg, or heart shaped depending on your type. That's okay any roundness or softening you get will make your face look more girlish. But just note that you might not get the perfect oval. And sometimes your own face shape might go inside the oval. It's not rocket science, okay.

Block out all the space between the original shape and your 'oval'. These are the bits that we are going to smooth out using our darker skin tone foundations. Figure 6 shows some samples. For each one the oval shaped face has been placed over the face type with the facial planes underneath. The area outside the oval is then blocked out to the actual face shape. Do not worry too much about the top of the head (see triangle and diamond) we can always reshape these with the appropriate choice of hair piece and or hair styling.

Once you have your own face map you might find it easier to achieve the next task if you enlarge your picture and tape it to the bedroom or bathroom mirror so you can use it as a guide. Load up a brush or blender sponge with some of the product one shade darker than your base skin-tone foundation. Gently fill in the zones identified in your reference map. These should all be on the outside edge of your face. We don't want too hard a line between your base foundation and this darker colour so blend it into to the rest of your face. Ideally you want a soft edge that transitions into the darker colour and gives the impression that the edge is round and falls away from the front of your face towards the side. Less product is more in this respect. Next turn to the darkest shade of your foundation and add this to the outer edge of your face where the most acute angles are and along the line connecting them. This is most likely the area just behind your cheek bones and down to the ear but also maybe a little into hairline at the top sides. Again, blend this into the colour of the previous step so that there is a gentle darkening of the tone to give the impression that there is more curve or depth.

The outcome of this stage is very subtle. It will go a lot easier if you understand the principles behind the planes of the face and use those as a guide to where you soften or round out the features. What you are doing in this step is giving an illusion that the plane is a slightly different shape to the ones that nature gave you. Go sparingly in these areas, not like a big ring all around the edge of your face. This is especially important if you have a rounder face. Confine it mostly to the sides and a little up on the temples. Don't' shade at all on the very top (or crown) of your face or under the chin.

Also do not make the fill-in between your own face type and the oval on your template too wide. Narrow is far more effective even if you stretch out or distort the oval shape a bit. A teardrop oval is quite a common female face. Don't worry if it looks a bit obvious at this stage. When you add your hair pieces these darker bits will look as though they are in the shadow of your hair and far more natural. What we are after is a gentle rounding of your face. Also, do not forget to fade it into your neckline behind the ear and just under the jaw for a more natural look. Whatever you do, always be guided by what you see in the mirror for the shape. It is a simple illusion but very effective.

When you get to the under-jaw area, blend so that it merges with the skin tone of your neck and foundation covering any concealer for the beard area. Otherwise there will be a tell-tale smudge that looks like you need a wash. If your blending here is a little off, you can always disguise it with a necklace, a cute little choker, a scarf, or a top with a higher neckline. It is important though that your skin tone and the two darker shades used for this blending step are not too different compared with your neck and torso. You might get fooled if you work outdoors a lot and your face is more tanned than the rest of you. If you look more Geisha girl your foundations are too light. Unless of course that is the look you are going for. If they are too dark you will look like you had an accident in a tanning salon. It will not be that bad (honest) unless you have totally the wrong shades.

The cheeks

Our attention now turns to the cheeks and for this we will be using the planes in the centre of the face. Remember a male cheekbone is wider and flatter than a female one. So what we want to do here is add some colour (or blush, bronzer, and highlight) to make it look as though flesh over your cheek bone is more rounded and sticks out more. The obvious (but wrong) way to do this is to apply two circles of blush right on the most prominent part of your cheeks and then blend them out. This is where disaster happens, and you end up looking like raggedy-Ann or the sugar plum fairy.

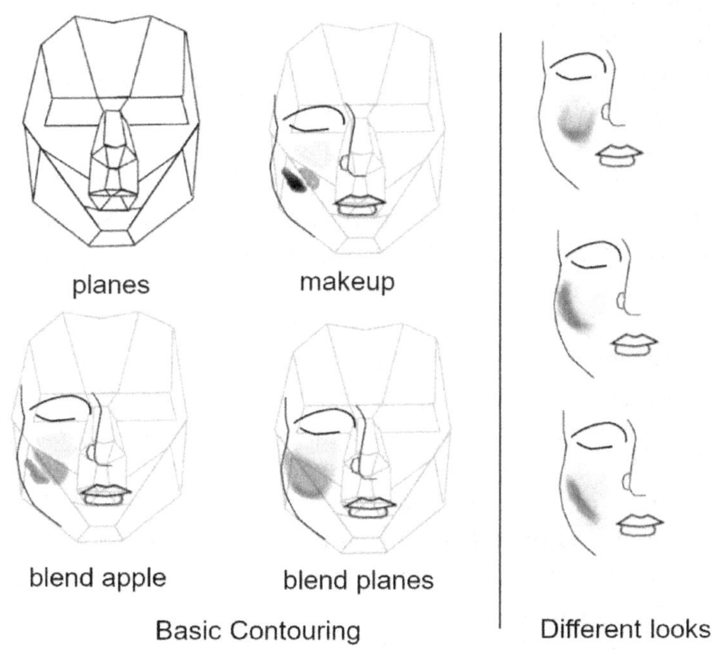

Figure 7 Contouring the Cheeks

Take another look at the planes of the face. Notice that out to the side of the cheek three different planes come together at a point which marks the change from the side onto the front of the face (see Figure 7). The three planes fan out towards the nose and dental cylinder. One just under the eye. One running towards the muzzle. And the third more down towards the chin. A way to find this apex area on your own face is to hold a blending brush flat to the side of your face with the tip on the top of the ear and angled down. Move it backwards and forwards till you feel the side of the cheek bone. The point where the planes come together is at this point where the cheek starts. Next, place the brush against the side of your nose so that one end touches your brow ridge and the other is angled past but just touches the end of your mouth. That is where the planes meet the nose, muzzle, and chin.

The apple of the cheek, the side cheek, and the undereye region are all defined by how these three planes project out of your face. Male ones are flatter and female ones are rounder. To get girl cheeks or a dramatic look we use three tones on these areas. Highlighter goes on the top plane. Blush goes on the middle plane, and bronzer or a darker skin tone goes on the bottom one. The combination or how hard/soft you make the edges of the planes with blending leads to all sorts of different looks.

To get basic (healthy looking) apples load a brush with a little blush. Start at a mid-point on the middle plane and then place the product and sweep it back towards the apex where the planes meet. Round it out towards the edge of the middle plane. Make it darker towards the bottom. This creates the apple shape. Make the apple curve harder or softer depending on the look you want. Use a softer edge and blending on the upper edge of the plane so it can bleed across into the under-eye plane. Add some highlighter on this top plane and blend with the blush so that the top of the apple looks kind of shiny. Do the same for the opposite cheek and keep them symmetrical. Experiment making the apples rounder or softer depending on the look you want. Rounder and brighter is more fresh-faced or farm-girl. More subtle is wholesome or girl-next-door. And just a hint complemented by a small nose is demure and cute.

You can give the apple more roundness by applying a bronzer or darker tone to the side of the bottom plane under the apex. This covers the flat plane of your cheek and is often obvious in men. Watch that Robert Palmer video again to see what we are talking about. The contrast between the blush/bronzer and the foundation is quite high in that video. For everyday makeup we need to be more subtle. Just give the underside of the apple you have made a little more depth to make it appear rounder. Alternatively, use less blush and a slash of bronzer on the lower plane to give a more dramatic look and to make the cheek appear more angular and diamond shaped for that Maleficent look. It can also give you a pinched appearance. This sometimes works well if you have a heart shaped or triangle face because it can make your features look foxy rather than little-red-riding-hood.

Use a highlighter on the top plane to give a little more roundness or definition. For example, this is like adding a bright spot to an apple to make it look shiny and juicy. Fade the highlight at the bottom edge of the upper plane and blend it across to the middle one for a soft or lost edge look. If you apply all three together then the contrast of bronzer and highlighter will make the apple (blush) part pop. This is because they are both neutral colours and blush is close to a primary colour (red). The combination will add some further roundness and make you appear warm and homey. But again, if you overdo it then you will look flushed, embarrassed, or maybe even a bit sugar plum fairy.

Okay then, once you understand the idea of planes and blending you can get more subtle. Most of the looks you see in magazines or on fashion models are about how you blend these three little planes and the product combinations you employ. Watch the movie *Grease* to see how makeup can give different looks. Pay attention to the way Sandra Dee, Olivia Newton John's character, changes as she goes from nice Sandy to raunchy Sandy. The other female characters also show a variety of looks from wholesome to everyday. As a challenge see if you can make your cheekbones appear to move inwards or outwards on your face. To do this move the location of the apex (where the three planes meet) up or down or further into your face. Alternatively, you can add width to a narrow face to make it look rounder by moving the apex out a little. Of course, to do this you have to be expert at blending and be able to fade into the side of your face. When you have mastered your brush techniques you will know how.

T-bar and I-bar

The next area of attention is the centre of your face which includes the brow ridge and the nose (or T-bar) and the extension of the forehead, nose, and chin (or I-bar). The letters are suggestive of the areas of the face they cover and since both involve the nose it is useful to separate them out into three groups (brow, nose, and forehead/chin). Some people prefer the T-bar others the I-bar. Depends on which of these features you think need more feminization. Be careful though because too much can make your face look over done. Subtle is the key.

Brow bossing: the horizontal on the T-bar refers to the brow ridge. We looked at this in preparing the eyebrows in the last chapter. Time now for a little more work. Depending on how much bossing there is this can range from barely noticeable to more Neanderthal. The best way to think about it from a makeup viewpoint is as a half tube or pipe around the base of your forehead. In fact, it looks more like the handlebars on a bicycle turning down on the side of the face. Have a play and feel the bump just above your nose and how bony your eye socket is just below the brow area and above the eye lid. That is all bossing.

The handlebar analogy gives you a clue as to how to deal with this issue. Just like a chrome tube the highest part will catch the light and then it will curve off into more shaded areas above and below. We want to bring out those shadow areas which means using highlighter. Apply highlighter to the bony parts of the eyes sockets and blend it into the side of the face. If you have masked your brows this will be over the area of concealer and foundation. Avoid the area where your brow is going to be. The highlight is intended to pop out the shadow area just underneath and just above the high point of the bossing to give you a more shallower girl shape.

The next area is the middle of the brow ridge where the bossing curves back onto the more sloping forehead and curves into the arch of the nose. This is the top third of the nose where the nose emerges from between the eyes (or nasion). The nose skin is thinnest at this point and both areas can generate darker shades because of what is underneath. If your forehead is more vertical (and so more femme) you won't need much along this ridge area between the eyebrows. But if you do, don't highlight the part of the boss that sticks out. Go just above to where the boss turns back onto the forehead to pop it out. Below the ridge highlight just inside the arch of the nose and either side next to the inner eye in a triangle or keystone shape to make it look shallower. Again, the highlight pulls any possible shadow out a little.

The Faux Nose: the vertical in both the T-bar and I-bar is the nose itself. Females tend to have smaller (or narrower) noses and the end (or ball) of the nose is often tilted up a fraction so that the septum which separates the nostrils is a little more visible when you look at the face straight on. The nose is mostly skin over cartilage which is why it is so flexible and explains why it flattens into a 'boxers' nose if it gets damaged.

There are four major pieces of cartilage in your nose and they all reflect light in different ways to give a distinctive shape. The dorsal septum connects to the nasal bone and forms the bridge of the nose before curving down to separate the nostrils. The upper lateral cartilages (one on each side) form the middle of the nose. The lower cartilage (again one each side) taper in to form the ball of the nose and shape the outside edges of the nostril. All this is then covered with skin. It is the dorsal septum that can give you that roman or hook nose. The lower cartilage can give you a bulbous nose.

The trick to making your nose look smaller and more femme is to know where to place highlighter and darker shades on these structures. Essentially, you want darker tones on the skin covering the sides of the upper cartilage. Highlighter on the lower cartilage where they come together to make the ball. And a touch of highlighter along the dorsal septum (or bridge) and a dab just under the nose where it turns in to separate the nostrils. See the section on nose tips for more detailed descriptions.

Now as we have said several times you need a deft touch. The darker shades make the nose look more vertical at the sides. The highlighter on the middle of the nose make it look narrower because it defines an edge. If you make either of these too wide, it will ruin the effect. And if you make it too narrow then the eyes will look bigger or out of proportion because the width of an eye is normally the same as the width of your nose. So, if you really bring the nose in you will have to remember to compensate when you are doing your eye makeup.

Although, wider eyes can look fresh-faced, if you like that look. Highlighter on the ball of the nose and just underneath make the end of the nose look perkier and cuter. This look is popular with pin-up girls and the barbie look.

Forehead & Chin: To complete the I-bar we switch attention to the crossbars on the I shape, the chin and forehead areas. Technically it also includes the lips but more on that in a separate chapter.

Men tend to have flatter foreheads that slope back towards the crown of the head. Female ones are more vertical and rounder. Looking at the planes of the face we can see that three areas comprise the forehead. The two outer planes to the sides of the head may have been made a little rounder when you made your girl face shape with the darker skin tones at the sides. The centre plane can be made to pop out with a touch of highlighter. Apply a small amount in the centre of the forehead (or middle plane) and then blend out horizontally and a little bit vertically. This should give it a more of a dome feel and work with your face rounding, to give the impression of a more prominent (non-sloping) forehead.

The bottom of the I-bar is the chin. Men have wider/squarer chins and females have narrower more pointed chins. The trick here is to make your chin look small and cuter. For this effect use a dab of highlighter right on the middle of the fleshy part of the chin (where the mentalis muscle is – see figure 2, in Chapter 2). Work it out in an oval shape blending into the rest of the chin. Don't make the area two big. Small is cuter. If you have a chin dimple, don't mess with it. Leave it free of highlighter unless you don't like it and want to pop it out. Likewise, if you want a little dimple or cleft add a tiny amount of darker skin tone and blend the shape.

By now you should be getting the idea that highlighter rounds out features making them look higher on your face. When this is added to your darker tones, they work together to give you a different face contour. Don't go crazy though. Pick the main features that are more male and soften them. A subtle hint often is more femme than a deliberate and noticeable attempt to mask something. The more you do the more theatrical or pantomime you will appear. Drag Queen make-up plays with the colours in these areas and creates lots of contrast. The pageant look uses much more subtle and lost edges to give the impression of smooth flawless but healthy skin.

Putting it all together

That is the next bit of your femme face completed. Here are the major steps again for easy access:

Step 0: Make a reference picture of your face. Add on your natural face type then sketch in the best oval shape you can. Place the picture on your mirror so you can see where you need to apply darker tones. Block out the area between the oval and your natural face shape.

Step 1: Use the two darker shades of skin tone to create your more rounded female face. Use the lighter of the two to blend into the face. Use the darker of the two to blend into the rest of your head particularly along the verticals. Fade in just below the jaw and under the ears to match the neckline.

Step 2: Find the place where the face planes meet on your cheekbones (the apex). Apply blush to the middle plane, bronzer to the lower plane, and highlighter to the upper one. Balance the mix of each to create adorable apples, an edgy cheek contour, a more chiselled, or a fresh-faced look with more highlighter. Experiment for the look you want.

Step 3: Decide which bits of the central face you want to adjust. Build your nose first (it makes it easier to see if you need other aspects of the T-bar or I-bar. Apply darker skin tone to the sides of the nose. Apply highlighter to dorsal (down the front centre) of the nose. Add in highlighter to the ball of the nose and just underneath for that lifted perky look.

Step 4: Decide if you want to reduce brow bossing. Highlight the eye sockets then adjust the ridge area between the nose with highlighter above and below.

Step 5: Make any adjustments you feel necessary to balance your face by applying highlighter to the forehead and chin. Remember, less is more. Don't overdo it with the highlighter if you have done a lot of work on the other steps.

Again, depending on your look and the degree of male features you want to hide you will need all or fewer of the above steps. Step 0 is a one-time kind of thing. Once you have made the reference you can keep it for future makeup sessions and once you get used to applying the makeup you won't need it at all unless you want to try different face shapes. Likewise drop step 1 if you find making an oval too much of a hassle or want to stick more faithfully to your own face structure. There is still a lot we can do with the right hair pieces and styling to soften your face.

Steps 3-5 can be used to varying degrees. If you are happy with your brow ridge forget that step or maybe just do the eye sockets. They usually need some sort of attention. If you have a rounder forehead or your chin is already round or smallish forget step 5. On step 3 you will find exactly what works for you. Some people don't do darker shades on the side. Others miss out the ball of the nose. Depends what you want or more importantly what looks back at you in the mirror.

More Nose tips

Like faces noses also have a few types and understanding how to re-model these will help with your appearance. Let's look at a few common types and possible features that people want to mask. In all of these remember to blend the shades into the rest of your face but keep the edges more on the harder side than soft.

Flat (or shallow) nose: in this case the bridge of your nose is not very well defined so the middle part might appear non-existent or place too much emphasis on the ball area. In this case place two straight lines of darker skin tone to contour the side of the nose. Keep the lines narrow so that the nose looks to have more outward projection.

Heavy nose: in this case the arch between your eyes is overcast by the brow. If you didn't treat this as part of the T-bar then you can reduce the shadow effect over the bridge by placing a small triangle of highlighter between the eyebrows and down onto the bridge to pop the area out.

Narrow nose: in this case the bridge is very thin and adding highlighter straight down the middle will make it look 'beaky' or sharp. In this case use two straight thin lines of highlighter on either side of the bridge.

This will make the bridge look wider. Of course, blend in or add a bit of dark colour on the sides to create even more nose definition.

Wide (triangle) nose: in this one the nostrils are much wider than the top of the nose. The trick here is to create a more hourglass shape. Apply highlighter under the inner corner of your eyebrows and eye orbit to create a flare at the arch of the nose. This makes it look wider. Make the nostrils appear to shrink by applying some darker shades at the base (sides) of the nostrils and on the lower cartilage that curves into the ball of the nose. This gives more depth. A touch of highlighter on the ball may also make the whole bottom half of the nose appear narrower.

Bulbous nose: a cousin of the wide nose is the bulbous nose where wider nostrils might also be accompanied with a more defined (wider) ball shape. The trick here is again to create an hour-glass shape to the nose but this time use darker shades at the top of the nose and as well as the bottom. This makes the nose look more balanced. Then apply highlighter to the centre of the bridge rather than the ball. This makes the ball look narrower and smaller.

Crooked (or deviated) nose: a common problem with noses is a deviated septum. This means the dorsal cartilage isn't straight so that instead of looking vertical it appears to kink to one side. The technique here is to use the darker skin tones to correct the angle. Apply two straight lines either side of the bridge. Then use highlighter down the middle. Ignore the actual shape of your nose. Use the straight lines to mask any wonkiness. Then blend as usual.

Irregular nose: in this nose the upper and lower cartilage do not join smoothly with each other or the nasal bones creating little dimples or protrusions where they meet. The trick of course (and you should be used to this now) is to apply highlighter where the shadows are to pop the feature out and mask it.

And finally

Once you master the basics of contouring and highlighting you can create all sorts of dramatic or cute looks. The whole principle depends on how we perceive objects from the light reflected into our eyes. So, yes, it is an illusion, but a very satisfying one. Of course, we haven't really changed any of your features so from some angles you will still cast more male shadows. But with a good use of hair and attention to how you hold yourself you can manage this at times when it is important.

Also remember that people have lazy brains. Generally, we do the minimum amount of visual processing we can get away with to recognise an object. This is called accommodation and it means if everything else looks right little anomalies will be ignored. But if something is out of place then it will grab attention and people will scrutinise it more. That is why subtle is best. Don't generate a tell by overdoing the tones or being cheap on blending.

Take your time and build up the colours. Be patient and each sitting will see a better and better face. Whatever you do don't try and make things look rounder. The shape emerges from the contrasts of the colour and will magically appear as you blend them together. Working from dark to light shades often makes the appearing contours more obvious as you apply the product. This will help you use the minimum material to get your look.

Remember it is all about how light reflects not what your actual features are. Do not try to paint on girl features. If you do that, you'll change yourself from Hansel to Gretal but you'll still look like a dolly. Work the product and go with what emerges not what you think you should be doing. In art they say paint what you see not what you think you see. That is good advice.

Chapter 6 The Eyes and Eyebrows

More must have been written about female eyes than any other part of the body. As one pithy maxim has it: *eyes have their own vocabulary – what a beautiful language to learn*. That is what we are going to do in this chapter, learn the language of eyes and use it to express your inner girl. That sounds like a tall order but once you break things down into the basics pretty eyes are not that difficult to create.

The first thing we will look at is eye structure and name the parts. This will give us a way to reference the various bits and help when we describe how to apply makeup and style the brows and lashes. Next, we consider brow shapes, how they differ from male ones, and how to find the right type of brows for you. Armed with that knowledge we will consider different ways of styling to get the right femme look.

The second activity will be all about eyeshadow. How to apply it, use eyeliner to create wings and tilt your eyes, then Mascara to add volume and pretty up those lashes. We explain how to use false eyelashes and ways to enhance your pupils and eye colour. After that we will look at a couple of techniques to choose the right colours for the best look and give your eyes even more sparkle.

The third thing we consider is how to cope with the dreaded hooded eye problem. This will show you how to modify the previous techniques for older looking and looser skinned eyelids. If this describes you then don't just skip to those sections stick with the preliminary stuff because it will help you in the long run. Finally, we round out the chapter with a few further insights, tricks, and tips to create some typical looks.

Eye Landmarks

Prettiness of the eye lays in the construction or configuration of the basic elements. Even a minor deviation from the ideal positioning can turn a beautiful eye into one that is well, meh. That is why women spend so much time on eye detail. A few cosmetic tricks can turn ordinary eyes into knockouts. Likewise, a boring male eye can become an attractive female one. All it takes is a few minor adjustments to where things appear to be.

Take a few moments to glance at Figure 8. The first thing is the labelling of the various bits covering and protecting the eyeball. Working top to bottom, we have the brow bone which should be clear of hair and which is usually highlighted (see previous chapter). Normally, there isn't any shadow placed here but sometimes it can be quite effective and something that drag queens and performance artistes emphasise. Next is the crease, then upper lid and the upper eyelash. Underneath the eye we have the waterline (where liquid gathers when your eye waters) and the lower lash line which is under the lower lash. On either side of the eye we have two corners. The tear duct on the inside and the outer V at the opposite side. All these places are where product can be positioned to enhance your eyes and make your iris and pupils pop.

The next thing to note is the configuration of the eyebrow in relation to the nose and eye. Ideally, the bottom of the nose, the outside corner of the eye, and the tip of the brow should all line up. This may not be the case if your male brows curve down the side of the eye socket. And even if it does it will meet the line closer to the nose than a female one. But if you trim the ends back you can always fix this alignment. The next observation is that the eyebrow arch should peak on a line straight up from the outside edge of the iris and sit on the brow bone (or above) not under it. This can be achieved by shaping the eyebrow. The third requirement is that the inner end of the brow should be aligned with the side of the nose. This is usually the case but if not (or you have monobrow), you can trim the inner end to make it happen. Even if the end is correctly aligned do not forget to trim anything that drops below the brow line. The thickness or thinness of the eyebrow can also be important depending on your look or the latest fashions and fads.

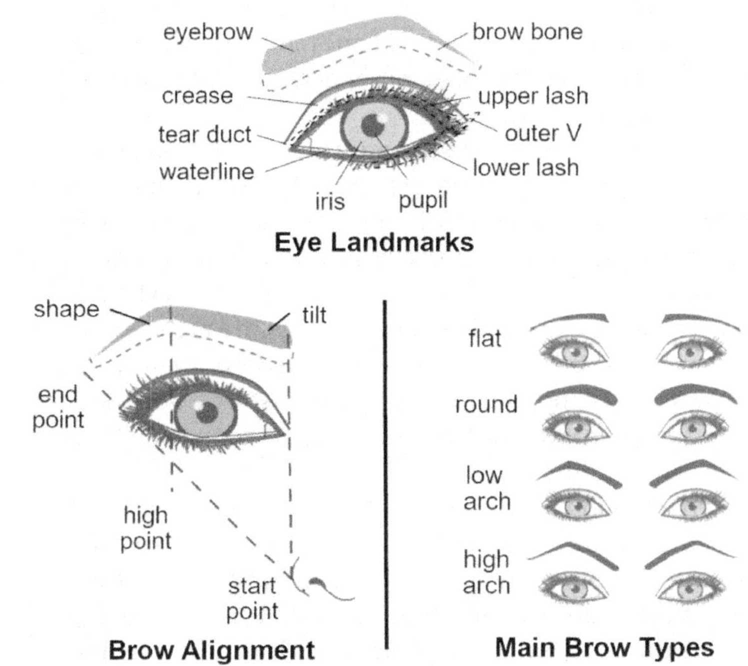

Figure 8 Eye landmarks and Brow shapes

Eyebrow Shapes

Now, before we get into the detail of eye makeup it is important to note that the right shape of eyebrow can complement your face type as well as your eyes.

For the three more female face shapes (round, oval, and heart) the brows are best angled. This means they tilt upwards as they move away from the nose. The tilt reaches its maximum arch just past the iris and then turns back down. The steepness of the tilt can be low or high or lifted which is somewhere in between. Softer shallow angled arches are best for the oval faces. A higher arch suits a rounder face because it makes the face look longer (or more oval). The lifted arch is more suited to short heart shaped faces and complements the inverted V (widow's peak) at the top of the forehead to give the appearance of more length. A longer heart face should use lower arches to give a more oval appearance. For male face types (square, rectangle, oblong) flatter rounder brows are better. In this shape the brow gently curves up and over the high point. This makes longer faces appear shorter and if the brows are fuller with a bit more of an arch, they help to balance a square face. For a diamond (or triangle) shaped face the rounded brow softens the more angular features.

So, now you can see the advantage of making your face appear more oval as we did in the last chapter. This makes it possible to use the classy higher arched brows without drawing too much attention to your face. If you use those arched brows with the more male types of face, you will look a bit like Mr Spock in *Star Trek*. An obvious tell. Especially if you forget to add the downward part of the arch after the high point and cover the brow bone with eye shadow. Even a thin and wispy downward inflection compared to the rest of the brow is essential to include in your look. Curves are always a feminine characteristic and soften your features.

A variation of the angled brow is the so-called S-shaped brow. In this shape the inner part of the brow curves down from above the brow line to touch the brow and then curve back up into the usual arched form. If the brow is thinner this can look very femme. However, if the dip down to the brow is too low then it can look as though you are frowning or upset about something. If the start of the brow is too high, it can look as though you are constantly startled or surprised. The reason for this is because these are the shapes that the brows take-on naturally when we use our facial muscles to make expressions. Having said that, S-shapes can be very femme, especially when they are thinner. Just use them with caution.

Feminizing your eyebrows

The easiest way to feminize your brows for real is to shape them into a girl style you prefer taking the above observations into account. To do this trim off any eyebrow hair you have that curves down along the side of the eye socket. This makes sure the first alignment condition is satisfied. Now take a highlighter pencil and trace out a line where you want the bottom edge of the brow (it might go across your existing brow). Remember to shape and position the arch in the right place to obey the second alignment condition (in line with the iris). Next take a pair of tweezers or an eyebrow trimmer and pluck (shave) the brow off under the marked line. This can be easier if you slick/comb the hairs down and thin out any bushiness first. Finally, trim the top of the brow for a pleasing femme shape. Decide how thin you want them and how much you want the curve of the brow to taper and then work out from the wider inner end of the brow to the outer end.

It is all easier if you have drawn a few examples in advance and know what shape you want. Before reading further take a few minutes to look at the different type of brows in Figure 8 and the shape of your feminized (or girl) face. Use a copy of your reference picture to draw on a few girl brows and see what they look like. Or, if you did that virtual makeover check out the brows that work best for you. If you didn't try it before go back and do it now. So cool to mix and match eyebrows.

False Eyebrows

If you feminize only occasionally or your dressing is a secret and the above steps are not possible then there are still plenty of options. Eyebrow and eyelash hair can get thinner as we age or because of hormonal imbalances. There is also a condition called Madarosis which causes people to lose all the hair in these areas. Although that is bad news for the person concerned it is good news for feminization because it means that the cosmetic boffins have come up with all sorts of ways to rebuild your eyebrows from scratch. You can do this if you have covered your own brows with concealer to hide them away.

Here are four ways to make the perfect brow:

Draw on brows: this technique is quite common because it is the easiest and most often used by females that have thinner or non-existent brows. It can also be used to mix up your look if you want to try thicker femme brows or a different curve. You will need an eyebrow pencil and/or powder (or pomade), and a fixer gel. There are also products such as lash growth serum if your brows are very thin or have been overplucked. Duo pencils include mixtures of products and textures. We will stick with the basics here consider the above if you feel the need.

Use the pencil to mark three dots for the inside, middle (arch), and end point on each eye. Check they are level and even looking for both eyes. Next sketch out the bottom edge shape of your brow with the pencil. Fill in the brow shape above this line with the pencil or the powder. In the former hatch-in the area with quick strokes so that it gives the impression of hairs. In the latter fill the area with powder and then use a slightly different coloured pencil to give the hint of hairs. When you are done seal everything with a bit of eyebrow gel or fixer to hold it all in place. It takes a bit of practice to get proficient, but you'll soon be able to create your brows like a pro. Don't worry if you smudge a little you can always touch up with a little concealer to neaten everything up.

Stencil Kits: if your hand is not that steady or you cannot get the shape right, buy some stencils. These are little cut out shapes that you can hold over or stick onto your brow area and either draw in the outline or fill the area with powder. Remove the stencil and then apply the above method to complete the look. Normally, you can get stencils in packs for multiple use. Be careful with the stick-on ones though. They are designed to go on skin not brows covered by concealer.

If you are handy with a pen, make your own stencils from some thin flexible card. Draw the brows you want (life size). Trim the card down to small rectangles and then cut out the brow shape. If you want the hand free to apply product use a small piece of tape to hold the stencil in position by sticking it gently to your forehead. Stencils are great if you want a very neat look but that is also their problem, they can look too manicured. Soften them a bit or touch up in areas with a pencil to soften sharp lines if it all looks a too angular.

Temporary Tattoos: are like those rub on transfers you used to get in bubble gum packs. They last a bit longer and women wear them for a few days at a time. The tattoo is brow shaped and you can apply them onto the brow region. They are called indelible but usually come off with standard makeup removers. Always check though. The length of time they last will depend mainly on the oils and hormones in your skin. They are less easy to apply with hidden brows underneath concealer but not impossible. Alternatively, or if you like the look think about having a semi-permanent tattoo. These can be expensive and will need to be done by a professional. Do your homework on providers and do not skimp on price. If it goes wrong or looks rubbish, you will be looking at it in the mirror for a long time and have to use concealer or the other methods to mask it.

False Brows: give you the most realistic look and are like little earwiggy hair pieces for your eyes. The brow is made from human hair (or synthetic) stuck into a gel and shaped. The underside is adhesive or will hold a glue so you can stick them on for a natural look. Again, these are designed to stick to skin and or thinner brows to give more body. Their stickability on concealer and foundation is open to question but if you have glued down your brows beforehand you can stick them onto that and then mask any protruding bits with concealer like we described in the earlier chapters.

When it comes to feminization, mismatched brows are an obvious 'tell'. They invite people to take a closer look. So, give those brows the attention they deserve and at least try to match them to your hair colour. Assuming of course that your hairpiece is one of the common hair colours. If you prefer an exotic colour or one of those bleaches like pink or metallic popular with younger females then just go with the eyebrows you have. And, while we are on the subject, if you have black hair do not use black to construct your brows. That seems to contradict what we just said but it doesn't. A solid black looks very stark in contrast to your skin (especially pale skin) and will make your brows look very sharp and false. We want angular but not sharp. Add in some other hint of colour with the black like a darker brown, ochre, or a darker gray just to give it some contrast. These are often called rich blacks and they help complement your features. The little tint mimics how your natural hair has variations of colour on the strands that catch in the light and helps to keep things real.

Applying Eye shadow

Okay, time for the bit you have been waiting for – how to get that product onto your eyes. Here is a generic approach that can be used with lots of variations to get the look you want.

Step 1 *prime your lids*: just like we did for the rest of the face it is a good idea to prime your eyelids. You can use specific eye primer, but foundation or concealer works just as well. Remember this layer is just so the other products go on smoothly and last. It also reduces the possibility of your shadow creasing or wrinkling as you open and close your eyes. Just dab little bits onto your closed eye using a sponge or your fingers.

Step 2 *choose your eye shadow palette*: We are not going to get into colour choices just yet. The most important thing right now is the lights and darks. For a four-pan palette you normally get a light and a dark and two intermediate colours. The way these colours are chosen is a bit of an art but the principle of applying the shadow is always the same so grab what you have and just follow along.

Step 3 *paint the whole lid:* we are going to use a three-colour (or shade) scheme. This is quite versatile and can be embellished or trimmed back for different looks. So first up is one of the intermediate colours on your palette. Load up a brush and then close your eye so you can paint the whole lid from the lash up to just under the brow bone. A small eye shadow or dome brush is good for this step. Place the shadow in the area indicated in figure 9 and then blend outwards to cover the rest of the lid.

Step 4 *apply the darkest shade to the crease.* Now choose the darkest of your colours. Load up a brush and apply it into the crease of your eyelid. Whereas for step 3 you will be better with a smaller dome shaped brush an angled brush will be better for this. If you don't have a crease, we will fix that later just skip onto the next step. The idea here is that the darker colour will give your eyes more depth and dimension, so they appear wider and bigger. The trick is to work out from the inside to the outside of the eye following the curve of the crease between the lid and the brow bone.

Step 5 *apply a light shade:* choose one of the light colours on your palette. Apply it to the bottom part of the lid as show in figure 9 then build up and blend all the colours till you are happy with the look. You might get a bit of gradient going-on and that is fine. Using small amounts of product as you dip the brush in the palette is better. You can't really go wrong with this but be economical with your product and avoid chasing the blend around your eye. What you do for one eye do for the other so they match up.

Step 6 *line your eyes:* take your eyeliner pencil (or brush) and draw a thin line across the lash line on top of your lids. Flick the end out at the outer corner (or V) to make your eye more almond shaped and to hint at a tilt (more on this later). Normally people use a dark colour like black for this. The idea is to make it appear as though the base of the upper lid lashes is a lot thicker than it is which in turn makes your lashes look longer and fuller. If you are nervous about using eyeliner or using a pencil use a darker shade of eye shadow and blend along the lash line.

Step 7 *coat your lashes:* the final step is to volumize the upper lashes to fill them out and give a little curl. Take your mascara, load up the brush and gently coat the lashes. Ideally just catch the lashes with the brush and then pull them upwards a little. The product is quite thick and will stick. The shape of the applicator brush will help give a nice curl. If your lashes are quite short you might want to use a lash curler to get them a little curvier before you apply the Mascara. Alternatively apply false lashes to get an extension (see below).

Okay, your eyes are done! That was easy wasn't it? There are more than a few variations and lots of style tips that will give you more than this basic look. Here are some enhancements to add to what your have learned so far.

If you find you aren't that good at blending yet consider missing out step 5. That gives you a two-colour scheme which is plainer but simpler to do. If you want an everyday look then do step 3 and miss out steps 4 and 5. If you do go all the way up to the brow bone this will allow for more dramatic or fuller makeup. For example, darker shades will produce the famous smoky eye look which we explain later. Use the first simpler look for when you are pottering in your home or at work. Use the latter for party time or socialising.

Consider using a nude or light shade of liner on the water line. This can be a bit tricky to apply, but it will make your eyeballs look whiter and wider or more alert and awake. Also think about a much thinner line of eyeliner or darker shadow on the lower lash line. Keep this out towards the sides to about halfway (just under or past the inner edge of the iris) and join it to your upper eye lines at the outer V. To top it all off just add a smidge of mascara to those lower lashes. This gives your eyes a more complete look.

Another trick is to add some highlighting. Take a highlighter pencil and just add a touch to the inner corner of your eye. The ideal spot is just next to the tear duct. This will pop out the arch of the eye where it meets the bridge of the nose. You can also enhance the crease a little more by adding highlighter just under the brow ridge. This will contrast with the darker eye shadow in the crease to give your eye more pop.

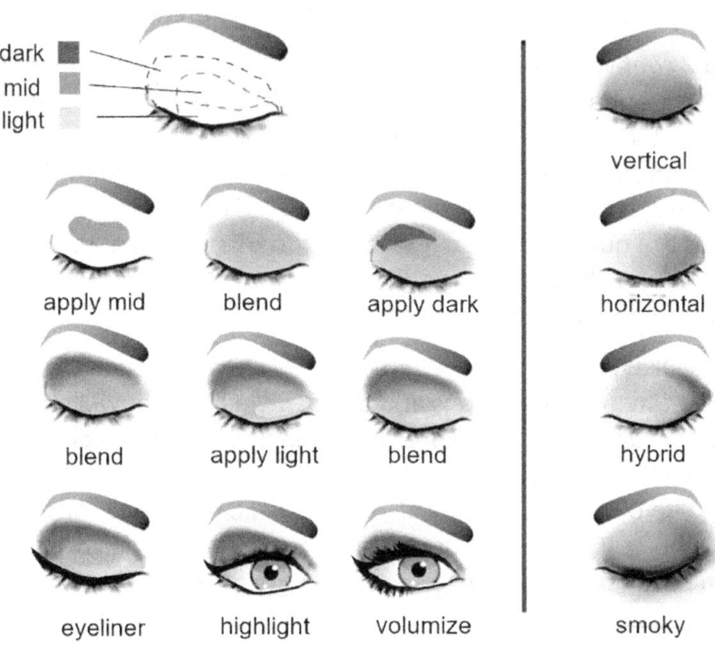

Figure 9 Eye Shadow and different looks

Developing different looks

You might be wondering why palettes have more than three colours. That is because girls like lots of variation and the chance to stand out from the crowd. You do this by making your eyes more individual. There are lots of ways to do this (and we will look at choosing colours soon) but in the meantime here are three ways of varying your look no matter what colours you choose:

Applying colours vertically: in this approach you take each of your colours (stick to three) and then apply them in rows (or seams) above each other till you reach the brow bone. Blend vertically to create some soft edges so that the upper lid changes colour from top to bottom. Always start with the darkest colour on the lash line and work to the lightest. This extends your lashes and also helps with the crease. Works very well if you have more prominent eyes.

Applying colours horizontally: in this method the colours are placed in columns across the eyelid and then you blend horizontally from side to side. Start with the first colour in the inner corner of the upper lid and work out to the outer The idea is to give your eyeball more shape so it is good for flatter looking eyes or not much lid definition. You can use the colours in any order you like to get different looks. The lighter colour on the inside helps pop out the arch. And a darker colour on the outside gives the dual effect of a more dramatic look and shapes your eye so it is more cat-like.

The hybrid: in this method you mix horizontal and vertical. For example, horizontal on the inner half of the eye lid and a vertical on the outside or vice versa vertical on the inside and two horizontals on the outside. The skill here is to blend them all into a pleasing contour using soft or lost edges. These can be effective if you have wide set or close-set eyes to get more balance to your face.

Any of these techniques will give you eyes some extra pep. The fun is in trying things out. Makeup should never get boring. Develop your skill for an everyday look if you go out regularly or just for a quick way to do your face. Then when it is party time or just for a change try a more exotic look. Eventually you will develop a go-to style and that will part of the femme you.

Eye wings

We kind of skipped over lining your upper eyes to give you a basic outcome but there are lots you can do to create devastatingly pretty, dramatic, or sultry looking eyes by using eye wings. The wing is basically an extension to the outer V of your eye. This can make them look more almond shaped which is seen as sultry and sexy. And, if you angle the wing upwards it will make your eye look as though it is slanted downwards which is another marker for pretty or foxy eyes.

A lot of girls get concerned about doing their wings. Mainly because it is a little tricky and looks best with liquid eyeliner which is easy to smudge and ruin your makeup. Relax. If you do smudge you can always take off the eye makeup and start again. If there is a little imperfection you can tidy it up with concealer or extra shadow. And, if you think you won't be able to match up both, it is difficult to get it perfect, but you can touch them up till they are not too obviously wonky. The art is to go slow and take time on construction.

Here is a procedure for perfect wings:

Step 1 *determine the endpoint of the wing:* there are two things to consider here the horizontal and vertical distance away from the corner of your eye. The longer the wing the more dramatic it will look and the more tilt it has the foxier. Too angled and long though and you are moving back to Mr Spock and too thick and blocky produces Cleopatra eyes. Remember the alignment of the eyebrow in figure 8? Never go beyond the end of the brow. A simple guide is to find the outside of your eye orbit (or socket). Keep the end of the wing on or inside this arc and it should look okay. Mark the point you want on the orbit with the eyeliner pencil as a guide.

Step 2 *line the upper lash with a pencil:* this is the same as step 6 in the general method. Use a sharp eye liner pencil and tilt it like you are using a brush. Make short strokes starting at the inside of the eye and work outwards to building the lining for the upper lash. One long stroke will pull the skin and the product will not spread.

Step 3 *connect to the end point:* When you get to the outer V of the eye draw a straight line to the point you marked in step 1. The line should be at the angle you want for the tilt of the eye.

Step 4 *make the wing:* look at the line you have drawn and decide how you want to link back to the upper lash. That is how thick you want to make the wing. Draw a connecting line or arc from the end point back to the lash line.

Step 5 *fill in the wing:* using pencil or liquid eyeliner. Pencil looks softer and is easier to control. Liquid though gives a nice sharp line and curve. Longer sweeps are better with the liquid and brush. If you really struggle with the brush use a gel pencil which has properties of both a pencil and a brush.

Step 6 *extend the wing down to the lower lash line:* this part is optional but if you also want to line the lower lid connect the endpoint of the wing to the lower part of the outer V (if it isn't already) and then sweep the line down under and close to the lower lash. Use the pencil to fill in as much as the lower line as you want.

Step 7 *touch up:* have a look at your handiwork and use concealer to sharpen any lines or to remove any smudges.

Et Voila! Now you have pretty foxy eyes. To enhance your look further, a range of common wings styles is given in Figure 10. Use the plainer simpler ones for everyday or work and the more dramatic ones for socialising. If you are dating or want that girl-next-door or even a preppy look use less dramatic eye wings. A mid style wing can add to your sensuality and create bedroom eyes. Often the change between your everyday look and your party or date look can help show a different side of your personality, indicate your mood, or add some mystery and intrigue. If you are more extrovert, then experiment away. Wings are one of the things that can turn plain Jane into a sexy kitten or a classy aristocrat. You might find that people respond differently when you do your wings differently. People that have been casual or indifferent can suddenly be attracted and interested. Practice a few styles so your can be sober, playful, sexy, classy or more bohemian depending on your mood

Here are a few more tips and tricks to make it all a little easier. First, if your eye flutters a lot making it difficult to get the pencil or whatever in position use your free hand to stretch the eyelid skin and squint your eye. This will put tension in the lid so that it is more accepting of the product. If you start dragging the skin either you are pressing too hard or it is time to sharpen your pencil. Remember for a pencil it is short strokes to create a line. For liquid longer lighter sweeps are best.

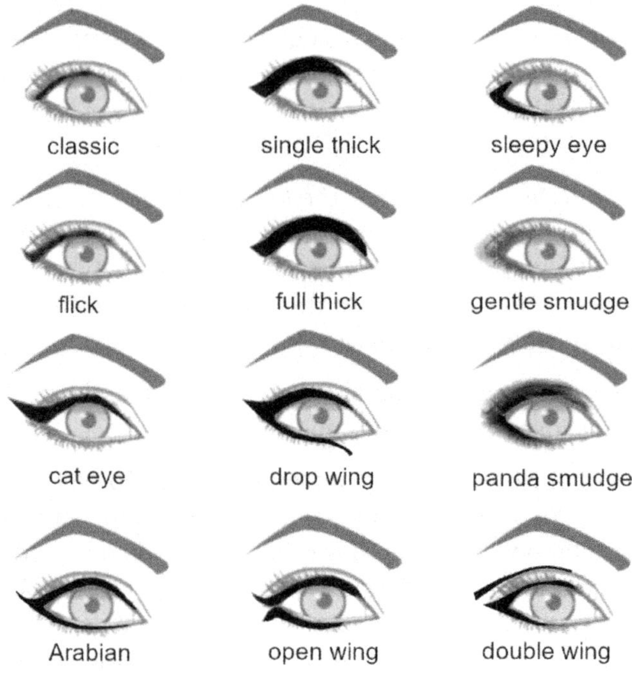

Figure 10 different eye wing styles

Black eyeliner can look dramatic and edgy but if you want a softer (preppy, girl-next-door) look you can use browns or other colours that complement your makeup. This will help bring out your eyes a little more and can be more acceptable as an everyday look. Also, if you are struggling with the extended flicked out shape a quick fix is to draw a # shape right at the corner of the outer V. Now just blend it into a wing shape with an angled brush and merge it back into your main upper lash line. Another tip is to extend the upper lash eyeliner inwards towards the tear duct making them fuller. This will make your eyes look more almond or cat like. The classic version of this is the Arabian style which is especially good if your eyes are rounder. Drop wings and double wings allow for a lot of creativity giving a more Egyptian, eastern, or boho feel with scrolls and other embellishments.

If you simply cannot get your eye wings to look right drawing freehand then think about using stencils. These can be bought cheaply and come in all sorts of designs from cat eye, double wing to fish tail (with two flicks or an open wing). Basically, you pull off the stencil and stick it onto your eye to create a template to apply the liner. The sticking power is not great, so it will not spoil your other makeup. You can also make your own versions but if you are going DIY it is better to use tape to create the shape. Choose something like the edges of those yellow post-it notes or art masking tape. Stencils are a good idea if you only want eye-wings for a special occasion or a night out. For an everyday look persevere with your technique.

Applying False lashes

The next step is to give your eyes more volume. That is to make the lashes a bit more obvious. Girls generally have fuller thicker lashes than men so this will instantly make you more femme. More lash will also pretty-up a female looking eye. However, it can all be a bit of a faff – so it is totally optional. If you do not want to have the hassle use mascara and a lash curler to make the most of what you have. We will also give you one or two other options below.

You can buy lash sets quite easily in the makeup store or online. The prices vary quite a lot so it is a good idea to know what you are paying for. First up is whether you buy a set of two or four. The most common sets have two upper lashes, but you can also buy sets with lower lashes as well. The upper lashes have the most volume with the lower ones much shorter. This copies the style of your natural lashes. The next thing to consider is how natural the lashes look. Thicker ones are cheaper but you get less lashes so they can be chunky. More expensive lashes are silky and thin and have a lovely light natural contour. Other factors in the pricing are the number of lashes (80, 120, and so on), the length of the lashes, and the amount of curl. All these things add to the look and volume so choose the ones you like and can afford. You can always add some curl with your eyelash curler so concentrate on the length and volume.

To apply the lashes you will need, lash glue, tweezers and some (manicure) scissors. Here is a four-step process to apply the upper lashes:

Step 1 *trim to size:* the lash comes with the hairs attached to a little strip. The width of the strip is a standard size so depending on the width of your eye you will need to trim it. Work the strip a little to improve its flexibility and form it roughly into the curve of your eye. The widest (longest) lashes go on the outside so use the tweezers to offer up the strip to your upper eye line. Note any excess and snip the strip with the scissors for a better fit. If you want more of the wider volume trim the inner end otherwise take it from the outer end. If the lashes are even a tiny bit too wide or have too much lash, they will irritate your eye every time you blink. Go easy. You can always trim off more if this is a problem. A slightly smaller strip is better than a slightly longer one. The latter will tend to catch or poke your eye when you blink.

Step 2 *apply the glue:* spread a little glue onto the strip edge. Don't go mad. Less is more. Just enough to get a hold otherwise they will look lumpy and the glue will show. Make sure you have enough on the ends of the strip. If this bit pops up with the natural movement of your eye it can be annoying and be a bit of a tell. Let the glue dry for a bit (20-30 secs) this makes it tacky and easier to stick on without the lash falling out of position.

Step 3 *place the lash:* okay, deep breath – this is the tricky bit. Pick up the lash with the tweezers. Look down and straight ahead with the target eye slightly open. This exposes more of your upper eyelid. Use a compact or a mirror on the table or in your lap. Plonk the lash on the upper eye lid near the centre of the upper lash line (where the eyeliner goes). Now shunt it into position with the tweezers. As close as you can get on the curve of your own lash. Keep your eye still and hold the lash in place for a few seconds until the glue sticks.

Step 4 *apply eyeliner:* let the glue set for a bit and then check out your new pretty lashes. The glue may show up in little clumps where it has squidged out from under the lash or smudged. Tidy that up with a touch of eyeliner to combine it more with your lashes and merge into any wings. A little wing in the outer V can help hide the join at the sides if you need to.

[Repeat for the other eye]

That is all there is to false lashes. Well almost. When you choose your lashes think about the activity or occasion you want them for. Lashes often come pre-styled so do you want that wispy natural look, extra curled, or ultra-thick. It will depend on the look you want and how girly you feel. Notice that the lash goes on top of your existing lash. Some expert makeup artists can apply the lash under your lash but this is a challenge and you run the risk of scarring your cornea or getting ulcers in your eye. If the eye gets infected and is not treated properly you could lose it. That sounds scary so trim them properly and put them over your lashes. Of course, if you want lower eye lashes too the process is the same except the placement is reversed. You go under the eye lash and stick on the lower lash line. The lower ones tend to be shorter and have much less volume. Place them close to the outside V under your eye. Often though they are much more hassle than they are worth.

After you have applied the lashes move onto the mascara step to give even more volume. You don't have to do this but it does help stick the lash to your own lashes, so you get more natural movement when you blink and so forth. Always apply your lashes between the eye lining and before volumizing (steps 6-7 of the general method.) Flirty eyelashes are a devil to get past with applicators and so on for shadow and wings. This order makes your life easier.

If you like your eyelash look and femme up a lot then consider making them semi-permanent. You can do this using eyelash extensions known as individuals or singles. This will also give you a more natural look because little clusters of lashes are applied along your eye line. This means that they can be positioned to give you volume just where you need it and give you a full and uniform look. The downside is that you have to glue each cluster on one by one. The best option here is to visit a beautician or an expert makeup artist and just sit back while they do the business. There are a few styles to choose from. A Russian lash is very fine and silky with lots of fan out for a princess look. Boudoir lashes are thicker and curlier for that harem or sweeter bedroom eyes appearance.

To avoid your eyes looking patchy visit the lash salon about every 2 to 3 weeks for a top-up. It will take about an hour and half for a full set of extensions to be applied (though half sets and corner sets are available). So it is definitely a girly day out – have a manicure and a pedicure at the same time and maybe a bit of hair styling. Your natural lash lifecycle is about 4-6 weeks. So eventually the extension will drop out but it is best to have them removed professionally using a gel and remover. It takes about 10-15mins. The good news is that with all that extra volume you can probably retire your mascara and possibly your lash curlers too.

False Eyelashes (and extensions) can be removed quite easily with a cotton ball or pad. Dip the cotton in some olive or baby oil (or any oil-based makeup remover) and swipe gently across the lash. Be careful not to get the oil in your eye. Wait for the glue to soften and then just lift them away gently without pulling too much on the skin. To clean the false lashes put them on a tissue or paper towel and swab them with oil-free makeup remover to get rid of glue and other makeup product. Do both sides. That way they will come up good as new and give you many hours of enjoyment.

Putting it all together

Now we have all the techniques required to do a good job. Here is a reminder of the basic steps combining all of the above.

Step 1 *Shape and colour the eyebrows:* your brows do not always match your hair colour but are tinted towards it. If you change your hair colour using a dye or hair piece different from your natural style try and match up the colours a little. Black brows with Blonde hair is a little out there and will attract attention but other colour combinations will need attention too. If you like, use a stencil or a tattoo, or other method to get the right look.

Step 2 *Apply the shadow:* using whatever colours and technique you decide. For example, single colour with a uniform look, stacked colours horizontal or vertical, or a mix.

Step3 *Line the eyes and add wings:* use your eyeliner to create extra focus on the eye lashes and use the wing to give your eyes a tilt or to make your eyes more almond shaped depending on what you want. Use a stencil if you cannot draw them on. Pencil is softer and easier than a brush but the brush gives better sharper lines. Touch up with concealer and shadow as necessary.

Step 4 *Add false lashes:* prepare your lashes (cut to size and add glue). Look forward and down and use tweezers to fix the lash to the upper lash line above the eye lash. Repeat for lower lashes if you want extension there.

Step 5 *Mascara and Curl:* apply mascara if you want more volume and to merge the false lashes into your eyeliner so they look extra-long. Curl your lashes more if the false ones do not give enough curl.

You can slim this down a bit depending on what you want or are happy with. If you feminize regularly then shape your eyebrows every few weeks and miss out step 1. If you don't want false lashes then skip step 4. Likewise, if you have eyelash extensions. If you do use false lashes then choose the style you want for the volume and the curl, that way you can avoid step 5. Plenty of options.

Brow stencils can be bought cheaply (£/$1-£/$10). Permanent tattoos are more expensive. A good set may go into the £/$100s. Eyeliner and wing stencils are around £/$5. False eyelash packs with multiple top lid sets are around £/$10, DIY individuals are around the same price. Salon treatments are much more expensive £/$100+. If you cannot be bothered with all the faff of gluing your lashes consider magnetic lashes (yes they exist). In this case you have two upper lashes for each eye. The strip holding the hairs is magnetic and you place one above your lash and the second below your lash and the magnets hold everything in place. We touched on the issues of under the lash fixing but otherwise they are considered safe to use. If you want extra volume in addition to the two extra layers you can apply mascara before adding the lashes. This gives you more hold when you apply the top one.

The dreaded hooded eye

Okay, that is all fine and lovely, except that maybes you don't have that eye crease to take advantage of and your eyelids don't make it easy to apply product. What we are talking about is the hooded eye. Here the upper lid skin is looser and so hangs down over the crease. The problem gets worse as we age. And it is more likely if you are male, fair-skinned, or overweight. They tend to run in families and scientists have found at least one gene that contributes to sagging lids. The boffins estimate that 60% of your sagginess is due to inherited factors with the rest due to lifestyle choices.

People get in a real tizz about hooded eyes but simple makeup solutions are at hand. The basic problem is that when you close your eye to apply the makeup and do all that work on blending the crease, it disappears when you open your eyes again. The skin sags leaving only what you did on the upper part of the lid visible. So here are some ways to make up a hooded eye.

Tip one: keep your eye open when you apply the makeup. This way you can see what is visible as you work.

Tip two: apply what we have learned about contouring and build a faux crease on the upper lid. Go ahead and just put a line of darker shadow on (your open eyelid) where you would like the crease. Use the brushes to blend into the inner corner and towards the outer V so that it looks like a proper crease. Do not make it too big vertically because you have less lid space to work with than a non-hooded eye and need to leave space to show the rest of your shadow.

Tip three: forget about using too much eyeliner above the lash. It won't show up. Use a thinner darker line and make a bigger wing out to the side. Also use longer lashes. These will help make your eye appear more open and hide the hood to some degree.

Tip four: apply some highlights. If you apply these to the inner and outer corners of the eye it will make the hood look more conventional as though the eyelid is curving in towards the tear duct. On the outside, the highlights help disguise the hanging fold. You can also put the wing on the edge of the outside fold to make your eye look more almond shaped.

Tip five: use different colour patterns (like verticals) to give more apparent contour to the eyelid. This will make the lid appear to curve over the eyeball. For extra effect use a bit of shimmer shadow so that it catches the light and adds more curvature.

Tips for Monolids

A monolid is typical of people with east Asian descent and are often confused with hooded eyes but they are different. Not all Asians have monolids but the majority do. A hooded eye is a double lid, the crease is just hidden because the skin sags to cover it. A monolid has no crease at all and it does not sag as much as the hooded version.

Monolids are just as beautiful as other eyes especially with nice full lashes but you can only bring that out by doing your eye makeup in a certain way. The basic trick is to use your colours to create a vertical gradient from lash line to brow ridge. With some subtle blending this can make the most of the lovely smooth curve of the mono and give a nice neat polished look. Also make more of the wings and eyeliner. Extend them up more from the upper lash line for a more dramatic look. Another tip is to use eye gloss to give your eyes a shimmer or sheen. This plays up the left to right curve of your eye.

Again, the trick is to keep your eyes open while applying the product so that you can see what will be visible. Some girls with monos still want the hint of a crease. If this is you, use the same technique as for hooded eyes and draw one in the middle and blend it to build the appearance of a double lid eye. The result will be variable. A better approach is to use eyeliner pencil sparsely all over the lid and then blend it into smoky wisps but with the heavier colour still at the bottom which looks like a little crease. More on smoky eyes below.

Colour Pairing and Other Techniques

We can't leave this chapter without at least touching on colour choices. How do you decide what eye shadow colour is best? Do you match it to your eye colour, your hair colour, your skin tone or what? Talk to makeup experts and they will spout all sorts of theories about how to get the best combination. Search online and there are a thousand and one videos for that ultimate look. OMG! Why is this so complicated?

Except that it isn't. What we are talking about is colour harmony. That is when you put two (or more) colours together they either fight each other or work together. When they work together you get more pop. When they fight, they dull everything. Or, one wins and chokes all the others. The effect of a colour also depends on where it appears. Is it partially in front or behind or next to another colour? These two properties are called contrast and context.

When we do our eye makeup the trick is to balance the colours we use on our face. A simple way to do this is to look at nature and see what works and what doesn't. For example, in a forest there are greens and browns and flower colours. Animals like birds are brighter colours to show themselves or more neutral if they want to hide. Blue eyes stand out from the neutral background of skin and hair. Brown eyes are more earthy and want to fade in. Green eyes are in between and hide themselves in plain sight like leaves on a tree. Get the idea?

Colour pairing: to make all this work we need to think of how to match colours. A good start is to restrict ourselves to just three colours: a warm colour, a cool colour, and a neutral colour. Remember that colour wheel in chapter 4. The warm colours are Reds, Oranges, Yellows and their combinations. The cooler colours are combinations of Greens, Blues, and Purples. A neutral colour cannot be found on the colour wheel. It is obtained by adding warm and cool colours together. The results tend to be more muted like Browns, Creams, and so forth. We can also subdue a colour by adding White, Black, and Gray which are honorary neutrals. For example, a tint is obtained from a colour by adding degrees of white. A shade is a colour from the wheel with degrees of black added. And, we get a tone by draining out (or desaturating) a colour until we get Gray.

Now let's think about the context of your eye. The iris and pupil sit on a whitish background surrounded by neutral coloured skin tones. Your iris is one of Blue, Gray, Green, Hazel, or Brown so sometimes a neutral and sometimes a colour from the colour wheel. Blue is a primary cool colour, Green is a secondary cool colour, Gray is a desaturated colour, Brown is a mix of a warm and cool colour (Blue-Orange, Red-Green, Yellow-Purple). Hazel is a Yellow-Brown or warm primary colour and neutral. So given our three colour choices of warm, cool, and neutral we have two of them already and pick the shadow to make up the third. Example, if your eyes are blue that's your cool colour. Your skin tone and the white of your eye are neutral so we are looking for a warm coloured shadow.

There are a number of ways to pick that additional colour:

Monochromatics: a simple approach is to just choose colours in the same colour family (Blue in the above example). For instance, we could just choose a blue shadow and vary the tint, tone, and shade to get a balance with the main eye colour. That is a monochromatic scheme because the only hue involved is Blue. Of course, you can do this with any colour not just one close to your eye colour. This supports the colour of your eye with extra contrast within the same context. It can be lovely but has limited pop.

Analogous colours: another way is to choose colours that are close by on the colour wheel. So Blue is next to the secondary colours of Green and Purple. If we look at tertiary colours immediately besides the Blue of your eye (say the two or three to either side) we will get a range of colours. A tertiary colour is one that is a mix of a primary and secondary colour, so that is Blue-Green, and Blue-Purple for your shadow. Plus, any tints, tones, or shades of those colours. Technically, Blue-Green is a little warmer than Blue-Purple because it is closer to the opposite side of the colour wheel which is where all the really warm colours are. Bigger contrast gives you more pop and the colour balance frames the eye with a different context.

Complementary colours: the problem is that analogous colours might still be too similar, so they still don't give you much pop. Pop comes from placing two colours together that have high contrast. The greater the distance between two colours on the colour wheel the more contrast you get. The furthest you can get away from Blue is by going 180 degrees around the colour wheel. That is directly opposite Blue. Since blue is a cool colour this gives you that warm colour by definition. In this case Orange. And if we look at the Analogous colours for Orange we get Red-Orange and Yellow-Orange. If we add in some tints, tones, and shades of these we end up with Pink and Coral colours. That maximises both contrast and context for your eye shadow.

Get the idea? As an exercise, choose some shadow for a green eye colour. Here is a hint - Green is a coolish colour and your already have your neutral (skin/eye white) so you want some warmer colours. Now try to pair up colours for hazel eyes. Hazel is a Yellow-Brown so technically it is a warm neutral colour. We are looking for a cool colour. That means we will be looking at colder versions of Hazel (monochromatic), Yellow-Orange or Yellow-Green (analogous), or Purples (complementary of Yellow).

How about Brown? Well the good news is that Brown is already a neutral mix of warm and cool colours. So we can choose just about any colour we want to make that third colour for our makeup. Decide what you want - cooler or warmer. This might depend on your mood or the occasion. If you want a cooler look, choose the cool colour in the brown mix and try analogous or monochromatic. For a warmer look choose the warm colour in the mix. There is no need to look at complementary colours because that is the other colour in the Brown already. Alternatively, use both the warm and cool colours that make up the Brown to act as complementary colours to give you two contrasting shades in your shadow. Brown-eyed people are so lucky!

Gray eyes are a special case because the colour gray is technically a mix of Black and White. Black and White are both neutrals and don't appear on the colour wheel. However, most people's eyes are not just a bland gray but usually have tints or tones of another colour, like Blue or Green. Check out the iris flecks. In this case you can go to them or a complementary to get a warm and cool colour to match the neutral gray.

Neutrals and skin tones: neutral colours can still be used to create contrast and pop even though they are more subdued. For example, white and black next to each other is a high contrast. Two shades of Gray will have more contrast as they move away from each other towards White and Black. This explains why Mascara is so effective in highlighting your eyes. The black of the Mascara and the whites of your eye set the context and contrast which pops out your iris colour. This is especially effective for Blue eyes. Likewise, creamy and nude shades can look devastatingly good on Brown eyes because browns already have their cool and warm colour combos.

You can enhance your look further by considering skin-tone and using that to help choose the exact colour mix above. For example, if your skin tone is warm then use neutral colours because your eyes are either cool or neutral so that gives you the warm, cool, neutral mix. If your skin tone is cool, guess what, you'll need some warmer colours (pinks/corals) or use silvery or blue in warmer shades than the blue/gray in your skin. And, again if your skin is neutral you can experiment with everything. That is why it is a good idea to get a honey or light caramel tan.

Matching to the Hair: If we widen the view, then the hair frames the face. Natural hair colours are also mainly neutral (Blonde, Brown, Black, White, and Gray). Blonde is actually a mixture of Yellow, White, and Brown. Red hair is not actually red it is coppery or a Red-Brown colour. That is, they are mixes of warm and cool colours with neutral. Black, White, and Gray as we have seen are also neutrals without any warm or cool colours mixed in. We can apply the same rules as above to pick out the warm and cool from the neutral hair colour to find a contrast for the eyes. Of course, this must be balanced with the warm, cool, or warm/cools in the iris of the eye.

As a rule, for Black and Brown hair avoid bold purples, yellows, or greens and if the skin is fair use neutrals. Red hair responds better to strong and semi-muted colours but avoid shiny or shimmery finishes. Gray or White hair tends to go better with pastels which are like tints or tones of a main colour leaving the focus on your actual eye colour. Blonde hair comes in a variety of forms from platinum and ash, through to champagne, strawberry, and dirty blonde. Because these have cool or warm qualities you can use neutral colours though it also useful to avoid dark colours because your hair will most likely be closer to a white than black. Thus, a dark colour with your light hair will create a background context that will overpower your eye colour making your eyes appear smaller.

Eye colour	Colour choices
Blue	Lighter shades and black eyeliner, corals, gray, pinks, orange-brown
Gray	Blue, grays, greens and more effective if you use a smoky look
Green	Muted colours work best – purple, plums, pale pink to purple, and purple-brown
Hazel	Bring out the primary colour in the mix - bronze gold or pinks and rose, beige and green
Brown	any colours will work but colours opposite on the colour wheel work. Lighter and darker neutrals like cream and chocolate have a nice look.

Table 1 Eye colour and Shadow colour combos

There is a lot there to take in but now you have the principles you can be much more informed about your choice of eye shadow palette. You can also appreciate why a balanced palette includes a neutral that will always allow us to tone down more strident colours and our overall look. If we use light (tints), mediums (tones), and dark (shade) colours then we can give depth to just about any colour on the colour wheel. And if we avoid using exclusively one type of mix like just mattes (which appear flatter) or shimmers (that add sparkle) then we will be able to balance depth and detail. Check out your eye shadow palette and notice that it always satisfies these rules. In a four-colour palette you get one light, one dark, and two intermediate shades.

Some Basic looks

Don't get overwhelmed or obsessive about choosing the right colours. The above will help avoid any obvious clashes that can be a bit of a tell. But go with what you like. If something looks a little garish then use the above principles to work out why and then tone it down a little. A classy or elegant woman or even that girl-next-door look all depend on mastering your control of colour. Some girls are just naturals and others have to work at it. And some, like all those red-carpet celebrities, use a stylist. That is the fun of cosmetics and why girls spend hours in front of the makeup mirror. To save you some time here are a few looks you can practice. Enjoy.

Romantic: for this use a base shade of shadow that has a reddish or rose-colour. Add a lighter top of a bronze colour. Highlight sparingly with a violet.

Sunset: choose yellow, pink, and bright orange. Layer the colours in rows and blend vertically to create the impression of a sunset going down above your lashes. Think tropical paradise. Don't paint it on like a picture just hint at the colours.

Earthy: this is all about neutral shades like brown, mauve, or a purple. Use your colours horizontally or vertically then pick out the corners with dark green on the outer V and use light gold on your inner corner for a highlight.

Teutonic: use blue eyeshadow with light and dark shades. Highlight with silver. This gives you a cooler look overall. Great with a paler skin, stronger femme jaw and blonde hair. Alison Doody carried this off to perfection as Dr Elsa Schneider in *Indiana Jones and the Last Crusade*.

Metallic: use colour-metal combinations. Gold is a shiny yellow, Bronze is shiny brown, Silver is shiny gray. For example, use a warm combination like rose and gold. Apply to one half of your lid (horizontal or vertical) and then finish with a darker shade of the metallic. Then highlight with an analogous colour like champagne or dirty yellow for gold.

Smoky: this is a very popular look that can use just about any palette, but the hint is in the name, so grays, browns, heather colours and any special smoky palettes. Apply a mid-tone all over the lid. Next apply a darker liner on the upper lash line. Layer a dark tone over the liner and blend halfway up the lid and out to the sides along the lash line. Smudge out (with your fingers) for a smoky look. Add some sparkle or shimmer with your finger and smooth out the lid to get a nice blend.

Smoky is not easy to get right. Which is why most girls want it. That and the more edgy independent look. The idea is not to have any defined lines around the eyes. It is all about smudge and blending, blending, blending to create super soft and lost edges. If you don't do that you'll look like a panda or people will think you have been crying. It is also advisable not to use more than three colours and keep the darkest point at the lash line (See Figure 9). Another cheat is to simply place your shadows all over the lid and then blend/smudge over to the outside corner for the smoky effect. Then add your eyeliner. For a really thick look use 3-4 coats of mascara or false lashes with extra curl and volume.

And finally

We are nearly done with our introduction to eyes and eye makeup. But there are just a few more things to think about. Females have all sorts of ways to send you messages with their eyes. To see just how expressive eyes can be take look at pictures of women with harem veils or those period dramas for that suggestive coquettish look over a fan or feather. So, if you want to be more authentic as female it is worth picking up a few eye moves.

Show your eye whites: we have seen how contrast works to show up and complement your iris and pupils so a way to get attention is to show more of the white of your eye. This is the staple of the fashion or sultry glamour model. The idea is to position your head so that you are always looking slightly sideways, up or down. You can practice this in the mirror but pay attention to where you sit and how you hold yourself. Always angle yourself so that you can look slightly sideways (this is called the three-quarter look). This puts the iris and pupils into one corner of your eye leaving the rest white. That is why looking over your shoulder is a sexy move.

Doe eyes: are flirty, sexy, or bedroom eyes that can look very earthy. They work best for people with bigger almond shaped eyes and brown or neutral eye colours. Think Bambi. Add some long silky lashes and a little flutter to the eyelids and you can look surprised, innocent, or a little overwhelmed. They are superb as attractors. It is often said that a woman can wrap a man around her little finger with the right look. Combine with the over-the-shoulder or sideways look and you are on a winner.

Soulful (or puppy) eyes require that you cast your head at an angle and slightly down so that when you look at someone your eyes are slightly raised in your sockets or pushed to the extreme corners. This shows more of the white between your iris and lids like before but if you also add a little pout, they become more puppy dog. And, with a slight downturn of the mouth become soulful. It also helps if your hair shades your face or covers an eye. This can make you appear vulnerable or shy and in need of protection which appeals to some people. Princess Diana was a master at this one.

Cow eyes: in this look you make your eyes wider, so it works well for rounder eyed people. Ideally position yourself lower than the person you intend to beguile so you need to look up. If you focus into the distance that will also dilate your pupils to give you a more passive and accepting look. Especially if you have full lashes. Don't overdo it though or you will look slightly vacant or brain dead. Some people like that Barbie and Bimbo look though. There is a lot written about maintaining eye contact when you are intimate but most of this boils down to appearing coy or submissive.

Flutter, blinking, and batting: on average we blink 10-15 times a minute. We blink more slowly when we are reading or using a computer screen and more quickly in reaction to external stimuli especially with respect to objects that appear rapidly in front of the eye, loud noises, or when we are dazzled or feel threatened. The normal blink is semi-automatic and the reactive one is called a reflex blink. It is thought however that blinking has other functions besides lubrication or protection because it happens far more than is strictly necessary to keep the eye healthy. By the way, it is an urban myth that women blink more than men. Women on contraceptive pills do tend to blink more often than other females and some women can blink twice the normal rate for men but when you average everything out it is about even.

One theory is that we blink more rapidly when we change our train of thought or as the brain switches attention from one thing to another. Reflex blinking, for example, can also occur as a response to stress, anxiety, confusion or emotional overwhelm. The staple of romantic fiction is when a woman meets an attractive male and flutters her eyes and goes a bit unnecessary. Anyways, a little harmless flutter will add to your feminine appeal. And, you might find your inner girl likes to blink more too. Don't make it too obvious though. Intentional flutter is called eye batting and can come across as a bit manipulative. These batting blinks happen 3 or 4 times slower than a spontaneous flutter so are easy to spot. The trick is to feel or simulate butterflies in the tummy to get a more natural flutter.

Eye flashing. A flash is the opposite of a blink in that you open your eyes lids a little more. An extreme version of this is surprise or concern. A practiced female can catch you with a little eye flash before reeling you in with some of the other moves. What a flash does is suddenly increase the white around the context of the iris, so it creates more pop. That is what we perceive as the flash or twinkle. An eye flash with a sudden look away can be dismissive or flirty. If you regain eye contact quickly afterwards it is a come-on signal. A bite of the lip or moistening of the mouth, a coy smile, a head tilt, or playing with your hair adds to these signals. More on that in Part 3.

Finally, we are often told as males that eye contact is the sign of a trustworthy and self-assured person. That is true to some extent. If you never make eye contact with anyone that can look very shifty. And, if you are always looking down then you can appear self-absorbed and nervous. In some cultures, though, avoiding eye contact is a sign of respect. And, averting your gaze can be seen as passive and accepting. In contrast, too much eye contact can appear as though you are drilling into people, singling them out (in a bad way) or being aggressive. This is especially true for females. At work or in the office then, yes, hold the gaze longer to stand your ground but do not give any of the other signals. When socialising, make eye contact briefly, look away or down demurely, then smile and look back if you are interested and want to engage with someone.

Chapter 7 The Mouth and Lips

This next chapter completes your face makeup. We will look at ways to give you a smaller and fuller looking feminine mouth. As in the previous chapters the trick behind this is the use of contouring combined with colour contrast. We start by understanding the various parts of the mouth and the surrounding muzzle or area. This will give an idea of the differences between male and female lips and how you can make them appear rounder or pouty.

We will look at the most common female lip types so you can decide which ones are the closest fit for you. The lip skin transitions from the more robust skin of your face and body to the softer skin on the inside of the mouth. Because of this it is much more susceptible to showing wrinkles or folds. It can look plumper and pinker depending on the blood circulation or the amount of moisture carried in the lip tissue. So, our task here is to learn how to control these variations and use lippy, gloss and other techniques to give you a sexy and sensual kisser.

Also, we will give you a routine to make up your lips, show how to give them extra colour, and then contour them in various ways to get different lips shapes. After that it will be time for some colour matching and how to balance your lips with the skin-tone of your face. There will also be further tips and tricks on how to apply your colours and highlights to get a neat and presentable outcome.

Structure of the Lips and Muzzle

The mouth is a slit in the muzzle. The muzzle is like a half-sphere that wraps around the middle part of your face just under the nose and follows the dental track of your upper teeth. We can fool the eye by changing how your lips look on this ball shape. The reason for this is that the mouth follows the curvature of the muzzle and a subtle foreshortening with contouring can exaggerate the apparent size and shape of the lips. If you have ever tried to draw a face this effect is what makes the mouth hard to get right.

Figure 11 shows a picture of the mouth with the major elements labelled. Study the subtle shading in this and the following diagram because it will be important later for contouring. The vermilion border is where the skin is often darker and fades into the rest of the face. Although we have shown a hard line around the mouth the reality is that the border is much softer and blends more into the skin. The tubercle and lobes are fatty tissue and give the lips volume and shape. Contouring the lips as they curve into and out of the mouth can also give more plumpness. Darkening the furrow under the bottom lip also adds further pout by making the lower lip appear to curl more.

If you have an average mouth the ends of your lips (or the nodes) line up with the pupils of your eyes. Male lips tend to end just on the pupil. Female ones tend to be just short of the pupil or in line with the inner side of the iris. The natural line of the upper lip arches up from the corners towards the centre referred to as cupid's bow. The highest part of the arch is usually level with the nostrils just to the side of the bridge of the nose. The way the muzzle curves out from the centreline of your face determines how arched or 'pouty' the lips appear. You can see that we are not talking huge differences between male and female, but with the foreshortening it is very noticeable. Just nudging the lips in this direction will make the mouth look more female.

Finally, as a rule, with your mouth closed, your lips take up about one third of the space between your nose and chin. The lip line (or where they separate to make the slit) is one third of this distance from nose to chin. And, the top lip is usually one third of the total mouth size with the bottom lip taking the bottom two thirds. Of course, these are ideal lips, you may vary around these norms depending on your lip type.

But if we can make up your lips to look plumper than these norms, they will appear more femme.

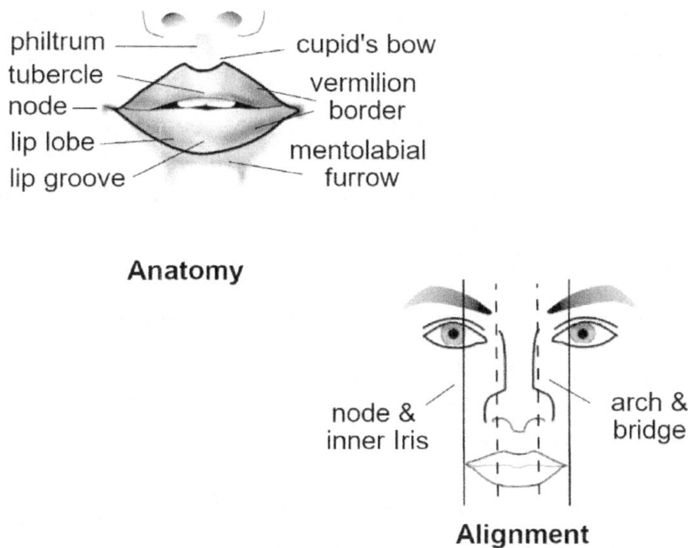

Figure 11 Structure and alignment of the lips

Lip types

Just like faces male and female lips can be divided into different types. Each kind tells you something about the arrangement of the natural lip line, the shape of cupids' bow, the corners, the tubercle, the vermillion border, and the lobe of the bottom lip. Figure 12 illustrates these main types. The most femme lips are shown inside the shaded cross. Lips are naturally bow shaped, so the top row shows what happens when you flatten or stretch the bow to make it longer. The middle line shows what happens as the lips get less wide overall and are plumper in the lobes and tubercle area, these are classic female shapes. Think of this as flexing the bow and drawing the string to shoot an arrow. The last line illustrates what happens when the top and bottom lips are asymmetrical with the pouty round mouth in the female zone occurring when the lips are again heavier and narrow but more balanced.

Here is a brief description of each one:

Heart-shaped: it will be no surprise that this the most popular female lip set. In his type the upper lip forms the top of the heart and the bottom lip narrows to a kind of point in the middle. This gives a lot of volume (or plump) to the lips so they look pouty and kissable. Personality wise people with these lips are regarded as passionate and glamourous. Rihanna carries this off to perfection with the right balance of fullness, plump, and shape. The shape of the cupid bow is also a point of attraction. For example, Taylor Swift is famous for this feature which she sets off with bright red lipstick.

Examples: Marilyn Monroe, Taylor Swift, Rihanna, Scarlett Johannsen

Bow-shaped lips: this shape is halfway between thin lips and wide lips. The name comes from the fact that overall; they look like a traditional archer's bow. Sometimes the bow can give volume and plump towards the centre of the lip. This means that the cupid area of the top lip can seem fuller and the lower lip lobe may be wider and more rounded. You can think of the heart as a kind of tensioned version of the bow (just before the arrow is released) whereas the traditional bow is more relaxed (before the arrow is loaded). In terms of personality people with these lips like to be pampered or the centre of attention so they may be a natural performer or a drama queen.

Examples: Kim Kardashian, Kylie Jenner, Chiquis Rivera

Round lips: in this type the upper and lower lips are about the same size but heavier and the way they arch up and down from the corners creates the impression of a flattened circle or oval. The flesh of the lip can still be quite plump and projects more from the face but not as much as a heart shape. Such people are said to be independent and adventurous.

Examples: Ariana Grande, Drew Barrymore, Jessica Alba

Full lips: have it all, they are nice and plump, but the extra volume is all over the lips to give them a rounded but sultry look. This type of person is all about relationships and empathy. They like to develop a close circle of friends and will want to mother you.

Examples: Angelina Jolie, Priyanka Chopra, Selena Gomez

Goldilocks lips: as we know from the fairy tale, these types of lips are the inbetweeners neither too thick or too thin, too pouty or flat. The cupid bow area might also be less defined. These people are supposedly rational and level-headed so if you need someone with a pragmatic view to balance your flighty side then look for someone with these lips. Natalie Portman has goldilocks style lips with a slight downturn.

Examples: Kiera Knightley, Natalie Portman, Sofia Vergara

The next set of lip types fill out the corners of Figure 12 and are a little bit more masculine. Compared to the more feminine lips they are flatter, wider, heavier, have less plump or may have some asymmetry compared to the ideal mouth shape and proportions in Figure 11.

Thin lips: for this type, the corners are further apart so they do not plump up as much. The cupid bow can be shallower or flat and the lips also curve less into the slit of the mouth. Sometimes the bottom lip can be very thick compared to the upper lip. If the situation is reversed with a heavy top lip you get a trout pout. These are typical male lips and are most associated with people with high drive to succeed but they can be a bit distant when it comes to relationships and may have a bit of an emotionless (or ruthless) streak. As we age our lips tend to get thinner as they lose plump.

Examples: Kate Middleton, Emma Watson, Jennifer Aniston

Wide lips: these occur when the corners or nodes of the lips extended further than the vertical line to the pupils. This makes your mouth look wider than normal. Because of this extension the natural line of the upper lips appears shallower and the height to width ratio is smaller, so the lips look thinner but they can still have a good amount of plump. Wider lipped people tend to be more extrovert and like to take on the role of leaders. They can be good at friendships but the downside is they can also be perfectionists.

Examples: Julia Roberts, Cameron Diaz, Anne Hathaway

Heavy Lips: The remaining two types are just variations on the above in which the top or bottom lip is fuller or heavier compared to the other. Liv Tyler has a wider thinner mouth in which the top lip has more volume than the bottom giving her a natural trout pout. Kerstin Stewart has a slightly bigger bottom lip than the top one giving her the hint of a sulky pout.

Examples: Liv Tyler, Kerstin Stewart

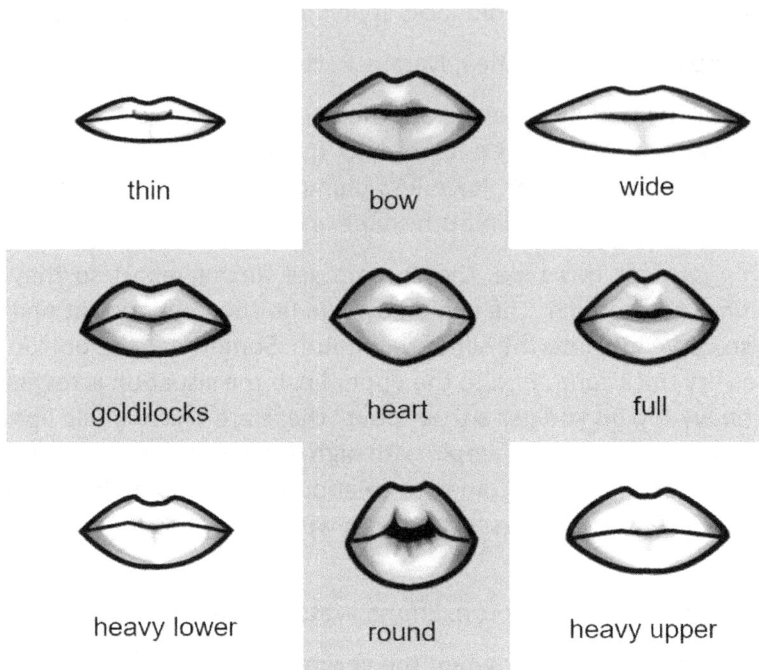

Figure 12 lip types

If you are intrigued by the personality traits associated with lips then take a look at Jilly Eddies, *Lispsology*, website (see resources). She claims to be the world's first lipsologist and you will find out all about the art of reading lip prints. Alternatively, try a Chinese face reading – and feng sui your face. Your upper lip is thought to show feminine traits and your lower lip masculine ones. Reputedly the shape and fullness of your upper lip says how sensual you are and your ability to love while the lower lips says how much you need to be loved.

So that is your lip types. Of course, each of these types has many variations so it can be difficult to choose a category. See how the tone of the vermillion borders help define the lip shape. The tubercle and lower lip lobe shades help to define plumpness. And just for the more femme lips in the cross some highlighting has been added to give the lips more pout. In the following sections we will learn how to get these effects.

It is a good idea at this point to see how you measure up. What type are your lips now and what type of lips do you aspire towards? If you have lips in the cross, they are already female looking so we can use lipstick and gloss to enhance your look further. If you have one of the types outside the cross, we will need to re-shape the lip a little first. No matter what type you have there are three female lip types close to what you have. Take a few minutes to consult with your inner girl. What lips would suit her personality?

Lip lining for classy lips

Lip lining first became popular in the 1940s and 50s. Hollywood actresses would use very solid pigments of lipstick with super sharp edges. Think Marylin Monroe, Janet Leigh, Joan Crawford, Grace Kelly, Audrey Hepburn and so on. Women of the time loved that neat crisp look and would copy it for big social occasions, weddings and for family photographs. Nowadays about 50% of the female population apply liners regularly with just over 10% using them daily and another 10% for nights out and dating. Solid lips are also the mainstay of models and beauty pageants.

If you look carefully at the outline of your lips where they meet the rest of the muzzle, you will see that the edges are not very sharp. The skin sort of fades into the lip and vice-versa. The greater the contrast between the colour of your skin and the colour of your lips the more defined the edge will be. The original idea of lip lining was to fill those uneven areas of the outer edges of the lips before the main lipstick was applied. This in and of itself gave smoother lips. The liner also acts as a guide so you can keep the lipstick inside the lip area and avoid bleed (or the spill of lipstick onto the skin around the lips). The greater contrast makes the lips appear to stand out more. Our next trick builds on this idea to ignore the actual shape of your lips and draw more girl shaped ones.

We can do two things to reshape your lips. First, we can shape the upper and lower lip on the muzzle to give them a less wide appearance by bringing the apparent edge (or nodes) of your mouth closer to the vertical with the inner iris. This creates a bit more of an arch up to the cupid's bow and so gives you a fuller poutier look. The second thing we can do is extend your lips outwards a little to give them more fullness. The idea is to go just beyond where the lip naturally fades into the skin. This is especially effective on the thinner upper male lip. You must be subtle though, otherwise you will end up looking like Lady Gaga in that *Paparazzi* video.

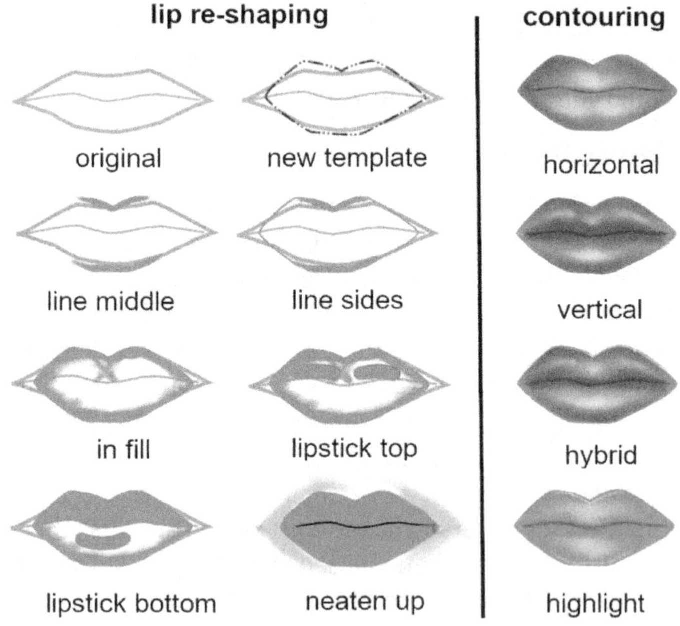

Figure 13 reshaping the lips (lining and contouring)

Before you dive in with the lip pencil it is a good idea to take that reference picture and trace over your lips and experiment with different kinds of shapes so you can get the look you want. Once you have the desired shape follow the procedure below to line your lips. Figure 13 illustrates the process.

Step 1 *Prep and Prime*: you should be getting use to this step by now. Gently exfoliate your lips and add any plumper (see below). Just exfoliate if you want to see the effect without added plump. At the minimum apply some balm to hydrate the skin and smooth over any wrinkles and then blot with tissue to mop up any excess.

Step 2 *set the centre*: start at the Cupid's bow and work your way out. When you get to the highest point of the arch (ideally just under the nostril) stop. Now line the bottom edge of the lower lip just in the centre where there is often a little line or depression where the two end lobes meet. This helps define the pout or bow shape. Don't press so hard that you are drag the skin, soft is better.

Step 3 *add the wings*: now continue with the top lip and draw the shape you want. You can follow your natural contour of your lips or use your reference photo for a more shaped lip to make your top lip look less wide. For the latter stop lining at the vertical close to the inside edge of your pupil. If you go for the more natural look then go as far into the node area as you can without smudging. Now match up the bottom lip so that the liner meets on both lips.

Step 4 *in fill* (optional): you will find that with a sharp enough lip pencil you do not have to press too hard to get a decent line. It is a guide. Don't try and make the edge too sharp that is what lippy is for. Some girls also like to in-fill the rest of the lip a little to help prime for the main lipstick. This avoids leaving a lip-liner tidemark when your main lippy starts to wear off. To get some fill press the side of the pencil onto the lip and smudge inside the line you have drawn. When you get skilled you can do this at the same time as step 3.

Step 5 *apply the lipstick*: okay time for the lipstick bullet. Apply the angled end of the lipstick and follow the contour you drew keeping inside the line. It helps if you open your mouth a little so you can get coverage on the inward lip surfaces too. Keep the top lip still and help the application by angling the lipstick bullet. Sweep out from cupid's bow to the edge on one side then on the other. Again, it is a soft touch, don't drag too much. For the bottom lip, start in the middle then sweep left to right (or vice-versa) to get the coverage you need. You can move your head a little or your lip to help get a smooth covering. Don't be too shy or tentative with the applicator. And, don't pet the outer lines, that will just invite a smudge.

Step 6 *clean up:* Nearly there. Unless you are a makeup goddess you are likely to have got a little unevenness. Neaten up with your pencil and a bit of concealer to get a nice smooth edge. Also cover up any of your lip that is now outside your new lip shape. When you get used to the process you might want to do this last bit before you start lining.

All that sounds straightforward but to get that pristine Hollywood or pageant look takes a little practice. Here are a few more tips and pointers.

Blotting: to make sure you have a smooth coverage and to avoid any excess finding its way onto your teeth it is a good idea to blot. Take a tissue and fold it over and put it between your lips and just gently press your lips together a couple of times. Any excess will leave an impression on the tissue.

Suck your finger: alternatively, take you index finger and put it into your mouth, grip it with your lips by making a pout, and pull it out slowly. Any excess headed for your teeth or lover will make a ring on your finger.

Use cotton buds: if you have problems with coverage into the edges of your mouth get a double ended cotton bud. Put it between your lips before you apply liner or lippy and hold it with your teeth. That way you will smudge the cotton bud not your face.

Use a lip brush: and paint on your lipstick. This can give you a smoother finish but takes practice to stay inside the lip lines. Using an eye shadow brush to apply lippy can give you softer gentler lips. This also helps with contouring to apply darker and lighter shades of your main (or base) lip colour.

X marks the spot: if you find it difficult to get liner and lippy coverage on your cupid's bow try making a little X across the area. This will prime the lip and make it easier to line or apply lipstick.

Smudge: if you think your lips look too sharp then you can soften things up by applying your liner and then gently rubbing it with a finger. This will blur the lines a bit. For a softer look you can apply your liner after the lipstick to touch up areas that look a little wobbly.

To avoid smudging your work of art during girl time use a fixer or gloss or use the waterproof and non-smudge lipstick. Leaving your lip print on a glass or cup can be ultra-feminine but you will have to be able to touch-up with a visit to the powder room. Otherwise you will develop a cheap look as your lippy wears away. One way to avoid this is to opt for drinks that have a straw or ask for one when you are out socialising. Sitting at the bar with your legs crossed girl style (one knee over the other) and sipping from a straw has a certain charm. Lip lining also reduces or eliminates bleed so that lipstick does not end up on your muzzle or chin areas. These things also help with kiss smudge but that really depends on how passionate you are when you smooch. Remember to air kiss when greeting people to avoid smudging them with lipstick or spoiling your own look.

If you are more mature in years, the extra paper/crinkle quality of your skin will show up the lip to face transition more. In this case you need to be a bit careful with the lining step. If you do extend your lips with liner it may look like you have just missed your mouth. We all remember grandma when she dolled herself up for a special occasion. We want to avoid the pantomime dame look. So, if this is an issue still apply lip liner but stay more faithful to your natural lip outline. Lips also tend to get thinner as we age so using a plumper can give more shape to work with.

Lip Contouring and Gloss

In chapter 5, we looked at how to contour to give you more defined cheeks. Now we are going to apply the same trick to give the lips more definition. The lips themselves point inwards and slope down into the mouth. Think of this like a thin piece of paper folded in half. The fuller the lips the more of a curve inwards you get. The bottom of the upper lip and the top of the bottom lip are more in shadow and appear darker. Also, just below the bottom lip is often a little horizontal cleft or groove. The greater the colour change in these areas the fuller and rounder your lips appear.

To take advantage of this observation you will need a couple of lipsticks - a favourite colour lipstick and some darker shades from the same colour family (see last chapter). We will also be using some gloss products, highlighter, and a white liner pencil. The right side of Figure 13 shows examples of the methods described below.

Horizontal contours: in this case first apply your lippy as in the previous section. Now take a darker shade of lipstick and apply only to the lip corners. You might find this easier with a brush. Blend in with your main lip stick shade. Use a slightly darker shade of lip liner just to frame the very edges of your mouth where the lips join at the nodes and the bottom of the vermilion borders. This makes the centre of your mouth pop out. The muzzle area appears more rounded and the lips fuller. With a bit of re-shaping with liner on the cupid bow and the lower lip you can make rounder, heart shaped, or bow shaped lips.

Vertical contours: to give more vertical definition and make your lips seem fuller from top to bottom apply the shades in rows and then blend. Apply a darker shade of lipstick as a base and then add a lighter shade on the top half of your top lip and on the middle third of your lower lip. Blend into your main shade and blot. This will give you a goldilocks, heart, or full appearance due to the appearance of greater depth on the lip as it curls in towards the mouth.

Au-Natural: for a more everyday look bring out your natural lip colours or use nude shades of lipstick closer to your actual lip colour. Add lip liner to the sides of your mouth to get a cleaner definition from the edge to arch of the top lip and curve of the lower lip lobes. Apply some white pencil to the centre of your top and bottom lips in line with the cupid's bow. Blend the white outwards. Now apply a clear lip gloss to give your lips an extra shine. This makes them look plumper and moist in the centre to give a more defined tubercle and shows the lip curve from one corner to another.

Highlighting: for this one you add some highlighter to the cupid's bow area to give the centre of the upper lip more definition and a bit of shine. Add a similar line to the edge of the lower lip in the centre. This will make these two areas pop out compared to the rest of your lips. For more definition and to make your bottom lip look fuller add a touch of bronzer just under the lip in the mentolabial crease between the lip and the chin.

Gloss and Shimmer: gloss comes in many types from clear to opaque. Some are so shiny that they make your lips look as though they are about to melt. Others just give a little shine. And some can have an almost glitter effect. A shimmer-flecked gloss will make your lips look plumper because they reflect natural light defining your lip curve more clearly. Although it is tempting to gloss your whole lip try a variation in which you just dab a little clear gloss right on the centre of the lips in a vertical strip. This will bring out your cupid's bow and the pout of your lower lip as well as making the rest of your mouth look less wide. Blend out to the side for the look you want.

Unicorn lips: if you are a younger girl (<30) and want something that is a little more out there try unicorn lips. This approach uses a mixture of the techniques above but with a wider range of colours. Think pink, purple, green, blue pastels (as in my little pony) and glitter or shimmer. Use two contrasting shades with one shade confined to the centre of the lips and the other out to the sides. Blend smoothly. Use a shimmer for a velvet look or a transparent gloss or even some glitter. There are lots of variations on this with a mix of horizontal and vertical blends or even a full rainbow look.

Gloss normally comes with a brush applicator, so you just paint on. However, it can be tricky to get right in the corners. Also, best to avoid too much shine where you have extended the lip outwards because there can be a slight angle between the lip and the normal skin which will show up more with shiny material. So a little trick to get the right coverage (which you can also use for lipstick) is to paint the middle part of your lower lip – the bit that sticks out more than the rest, and then just rub your lips together to spread it outwards onto the rest of your mouth.

Experiment with the above approaches until you find the balance that works for you. For example, you might find that you mix a vertical contour with just a hint of highlighting. Alternatively, you might like a smoother satin feel to the lips rather than a full-on gloss. You might try a toned version for everyday and then jazz up a little for party time. If you want to be a little more dramatic but not the full unicorn, apply the same principle but with lipstick shades from your preferred colour family.

Colour choices and matching

You can get a wide range of looks from the dramatic femme fatale to the natural ingenue with the right choice of lip colour. But which colours go with what? Remember all that colour theory in the last chapter? Well it applies here too. You can match your lipstick to your skin-tone, eyes, or hair colours. Skin as we pointed out before is a neutral colour so use your skin under tone to pick out a colour for your lippy. The white of the teeth also create contrast with the lip as it darkens and turns into the mouth.

For cooler undertones use lipsticks which have a balance of blue or purple in the mix. Not necessarily that as the main colour just a tint or tone to the base colour you want. Deeper reds and pinks will also work if you want more contrast. If you have a warm undertone it is corals and orangey hues. Bright red will work well on you and nudes will also look good. For the neutral under tone, again you can get away with just about any shade, but it may payoff more to match your eye and hair colour. One rule for any skin tone is that if your lips are thin avoid darker lipsticks. They will just make your lips look even thinner.

To match your lipstick with your hair again look at the undertones. No one really has a uniform hair colour so see how it catches the light and notice the tints and tones. For example, if you have blonde hair it might have golden, ashy, or brown elements. If you are a red head then does it have hotter redder elements, cooler reds, or copper. And for brunettes you have a whole range of browns and darks. Match these colours with the tones and tints in your lipstick. Black hair goes well with reds particularly rose/pink and shades a few tones darker than your own lips. For Gray or white hair the best option is to go for nude colours or your natural lip colour. Match the liner and then use a sheer nude or pink gloss for a softer natural look. If you do want colour than use a red with a blue base, corals and berry shades like strawberry and raspberry.

Now, every girl wants to try red. Red lipstick has a long and fascinating history and is seen as the most powerful expression of female beauty and sexuality. It will work on just about anyone (except perhaps for very thin lips when it is a bit Cruella De Vil). The trick is to choose the right tone of red. A general rule is the lighter your hair and eye colour choose more orange reds. Deeper (berry) reds work better for darker eye and hair colours. Check out Sean Young, as Rachel, in the hit film *Bladerunner* for an almost perfect balance of makeup with red lipstick. Likewise, Taylor swift wears red lippy really well. And Rihanna excels with more velvety plum colours.

The darker shades of lipstick tend to have a more vampire like effect. Good if you like Goth but they can make you look a little scary and/or older. A comprise is to use a berry colour which has a hint of red which adds a bit of sensuality. A very strident and bold red is often the staple of the more assured or dominant lady, but it can also be a bit tarty – as in the French Bordello look. That overly red lipstick is seen as risqué because it mimics the arousal and rush of blood to your, ahem, lady bits. Apparently, the juxtaposition of these two extremes, the thing you lust after but cannot have, drives some guys nuts. So, if you wear red be prepared to have a withering put down or a sexy line ready. For some classy bordello looks check out the French TV series *Maison Close*.

Pink lips come in and out of fashion. A subtle pink can look very femme and is a staple of the 'preppy' look. But do be careful. Bubble-gum pink has a bit of a reputation. It is the staple of porn actresses and seen as a 'barbie' colour by many people. That might sound harsh, but if you want to avoid getting the ditsy bimbo label go for more rosy-red hints of red or the corals. Back off on the lip plump the pinker you go. Then again, if ditsy and cute is the thing you are after, go for it. Bubble-gum is great with a high gloss and odango hair if you have a sissy gurl persona. Gwen Stefani does a good nude makeup look and also manages pink and red lippy very well if you want a classier look.

The beige and cream (or nude) colours are great for an everyday or understated but refined look. They work well with brunettes. Choose a shade that is a little darker or slightly brighter than your skin tone. If you go too dark your face will look pale and pasty. Too light and you lose all that lip definition and your lips fade into the rest of your face. Nude always looks good with a little gloss or shimmer. The two girls in the band ABBA were masters at this technique -check out some of their music videos to get the look.

Lip plumping

A major element of fuller lips is the amount of plump. As a rule, female lips are more plumped than male ones. The male upper lip can be especially thin. So, how do we give those lips an extra bit of volume without visiting the plastic surgeon? The lips are capable of changing size quite dramatically as a reaction to your state of excitement, changes in temperature, the amount of hydration, as well as allergies. When they are cold or under hydrated, they can shrink and wrinkle up. When they are hot, the body is jazzed with anticipation, or your heart is beating faster they will swell and stretch the skin giving them a smooth fuller appearance. That is why fuller lips are considered sexy and sensual because they often indicate excitement or arousal.

Fortunately, there are lots of ways to plump your lips naturally. Here are a few of the most popular methods that will result in a temporary plump for a few hours or so. This is ideal for occasional feminization and gives plenty of time for camming or to take selfies and so on.

Exfoliation: the first method relies on the ability of the lips to react to mild irritation as a result the lips will appear plumper for a short time. The trick is to rub your lips gently with a dry toothbrush. This will take off any dead skin cells making the lip surface smoother. And the stimulation will improve blood flow and circulation which will make the lip swell a little. If you want a more sensuous look add some honey or a little bit of Vaseline to the toothbrush which will make the skin even smoother and give your lips a naturally pinker tone.

Scrubs: a variant on the above is to make up a simple scrub using a mix of sugar and water. Make a thin paste and then add a few drops of moisturizing oil. Apply the scrub to your lips and massage it around in small circles. The coarseness of the sugar will exfoliate and mildly irritate the skin but the effect should quickly disappear. The oil will penetrate the skin and act as a hydrator giving you a bit more volume for a longer period.

Essential Oils: can be used with other common ingredients to make a version of the lip-plumpers you can buy from cosmetic shops, beauty parlours and drug stores. The effect does not last as long as a purpose made plumper but will be good for a few hours. The idea is that you add a small drop of a chosen oil to your lip balm. Less is more, trust me. Then all you do is apply the lip balm and you are good to go. The oil stimulates and widens the capillaries in the lips increasing blood flow so that you get fuller lips with an extra rosy effect because of the extra blood under the skin. A bonus is that the oil will give you a more girly aroma. You should feel a mild tingling (or burning) sensation for a few minutes and then it will disappear. Wash everything off immediately, if the sensation doesn't disappear, or your lips swell dramatically.

Celebrity mixes appear quite regularly so if you admire the lips of a particular starlet or model see what mix she uses. A popular one is Cinnamon, Cayenne pepper, and Coconut oil. Apply the mix to your lips and then just dab off and wait for the tingling to subside and leave you with fuller lips. The coconut oil makes your lips softer and more kissable. It is important to balance the ingredients though. Other popular choices of oil include Peppermint which brings blood closer to surface giving a bit more swell and adds a cooling effect. Do not get Cayenne pepper oil. confused with ground Cayenne pepper powder. The latter can be mixed with water in very very tiny amounts and rubbed on the lips for more plump. If you over do it (which is real easy) it will sting and burn like crazy.

Hyaluronic acid: is the staple of many of the over the counter plumpers. The main ingredient acts as a deep moisturizer which penetrates the lips to give them a fuller appearance. The extra fluid makes the plump last for much longer than the previous methods and some products also come with sun protection, so they are good if you want to go out while you are en-femme. Hyaluronic acid is a type of sugar found in your connective tissues, joints, and skin. It helps keep your skin supple and firm. Its other main property is that it can hold up to 1,000 times its weight in water. Because it is already in your body it is unlikely to cause an allergic reaction. This makes it a good choice for plumping.

Vacuum Plumping: next up is using suction to increase the blood flow into the lips giving them more volume and that reddish appearance. This method will give up to 10 hours of extra plump and with regular use maybe a little longer. The principle is the same as cupping, where you heat up something like a glass or cup and then place the rim on the skin. As the trapped air cools, it forms a vacuum and draws skin upwards into the cup. The skin and blood vessels underneath will turn redder as they react to the pressure difference and expand. There are celebrity tales of people using shot glasses on their lips in this way but this is not to be recommended because (apart from the danger of breaking the glass and cutting your lip) you have to apply them several times and might get a variable plump across the lips. Electronic stimulators and suction devices made specially for the lips can be bought relatively cheaply in stores or on-line. The results can be variable though and depend on skin sensitivity and lip shape. You might also experience some bruising.

Lip exercises: this final method will give you the most long-lasting effect but takes time and dedication. Did you ever notice that people that play musical instruments requiring use of the mouth tend to have fuller lips? The principle is that the constant pouting, sucking, and blowing on the instrument is like a workout for your lips and builds up collagen for a more natural plump. Limber up your lips everyday with some pouting, (air) kissing, or whistling. Smile really widely and hold it for a few seconds then air kiss and hold that for a few seconds. Repeat this 20-30 times every day for a couple of months and your lips will firm up. Alternatively, take up music and learn to play a wind instrument. The most popular choices for girls are the flute, clarinet, and oboe.

It probably goes without saying that you should not over plump your lips. Apart from looking like a bit of a lush, when the lip swells too much the inside is pulled outwards and the sensitive tissue dries out. Do this regularly and you may end with cracked lips. If your lips itch or start to look like a bee sting or the lips continue to burn, or you get little red patches, or a rash then clean off the plumper immediately. Throw away that product or do not repeat the mix you used or stick with contouring.

Anyways, if this is your thing, you have a choice of methods depending on what you want to achieve. The best approach is to apply your method and then wait for 5-10mins for the reaction to take place and for the lips to swell. After that apply a lipstick or gloss and you are good to go. For a more natural look just apply a lip balm or gloss and let your natural lip colour show through.

Putting it all together

Okay, time to summarise and throw it all together into your lip routine.

Step 1 *prepare the lips:* that is exfoliate and hydrate- make this part of your normal girl time pamper routine and you will not have to do much at makeup time.

Step 2 *plump:* apply a plumping technique to give the lips a little swell and boost blood circulation. You will need to wait 5-10mins for things to take effect. These first two steps prime your lips.

Step 3 *choose your colours:* while you are waiting for the plump to take effect pick out your colours and decide how you are going to apply them.

Step 4 *line the lips*: apply the lip pencil to get the desired shape and definition. Follow your natural line if you are happy with your mouth size. Otherwise, re-draw the lip for a different/smaller look.

Step 5 *base lipstick*: apply your base lipstick. Work out from the centre on the top lip and sweep back and forth on the bottom one. If you are not interested in contouring skip the next step.

Step 6 *contour*: use your other lipstick colours to add further curve and volume to the lips using one of the techniques (vertical, horizontal etc) in the previous section. Apply them with a brush for more precision and for blending.

Step 7 *touch-up*: check for neatness and crisp lines if that is your look. Apply any concealer or lip pencil to straighten and cover over wobbles and any lip skin now outside your new lip contour.

Step 8 *highlight and gloss*: finish off with a coat of gloss to give you some extra curve to the lips. Highlight cupid's bow and lower lip as necessary. Add bronzer just under the bottom lip.

That is the full procedure but your might want to play with the steps and skip some depending on what you see in the mirror as you work. If all you want is a quick fix with a bit of plump and shine go with your natural colours and steps 1, 2, and 8. If you don't like the idea of irritating your skin skip step 2 and use step 6 to get more definition. If you want that Hollywood starlet look skip the gloss section. Go with steps 4, 5, and 7 using a solid pigment lipstick with a bit of a satin or matte look. It really is up to you.

And finally

That is just about it for your lips and mouth. Just a few more little observations that you might find helpful.

First, if your normal lip colour is a bit patchy or they look bruised, cover up with some concealer to nude out before you start applying the lipstick. This will give a nice even tone. A solid pigment should cover everything, but if you are gloss only or using more natural colours like nudes, the right concealer will save the day. If your lips are very thin and you have trouble applying the products try using a brush. Gloss has a brush applicator as do liquid lipsticks. The bullet forms are quite greasy and melt easily so you can use a small makeup brush to apply your lipstick in those hard to reach areas. Also, if your upper lip is very thin the gap between your nose and lip might seem quite large. Do not try and make all this up with higher lip lining. Add some bronzer just under your nose to give more of a shadow effect there which will reduce the apparent distance and then work with a more natural lip line to make the mouth appear closer to your nose and more femme.

If you are dolling-it-up for some intimate play it follows that you are not going to stay looking pristine. You might like that used look but if not replace your lipstick with a lip stain. A stain is a lightweight, glossy, and watery mix. What you get is the deposit of pigment but not much texture. That will make your lips bolder but otherwise leave them in a natural state. Stains are pretty much like the ancient technique of biting a berry to colour your lips with juice. The stain does what it says and does not sit on top of the lip like other products. This means it is long lasting and wears away slowly. Also, it will not melt if you are somewhere hot. You can remove the colour quite easily with cleanser. Anyhow, if this is relevant to you or you cannot be bothered with all the rigmarole above then consider a stain.

Finally, it goes without saying, when you are out and about keep your mitts off your face. If you are a toucher and like to rub your eyes, your nose, touch your lips, or heaven forbid, bite your fingernails, all you will do is smudge everything and ruin your hard work. More to the point you will become an object of interest for on-lookers and once they look closely, they may start wonder. So, if you really are Miss Fidget, find a distractor. Use a compact, sit on your hands, use your phone, or keep them otherwise occupied. Holding hands lightly in your lap is a nice and femme thing to do when you have an idle moment. Even playing with a strand of hair can be cute. But no face touching, okay.

Part 3
Hair and Hair styling

"Hair doesn't make the woman, but good hair definitely helps."

– Unknown

"Hair style is the final tip-off whether or not a woman really knows herself."

– Hubert de Givenchy

Chapter 8 Hair Pieces, Accessories, and more

The next few chapters will introduce you to all the things that females do with their hair. Some of this will be functional, to allow you to manage more volume of hair than you are perhaps used to. Some things will be social as in how to express your female personality and understand the expectations of others. And, some things will be about fashion trends and an ideal female look. A further objective is to give you the vocabulary of hair management and style. This is an important aspect of your socialisation. It will allow us to quickly describe different looks and for you to girl talk knowledgeably with your friends. Together all these things will make you more authentic.

One reason for thinking about hair pieces is that as men age the hair tends to get thinner. Pattern baldness such as a receding hair line or a bald patch can appear. By the age of thirty about 25% of men have started to go bald and by forty-five that is more like 50%. And, overall, 80% of men have some hair loss as they age. In fact, you do not actually lose hair, you have the same number of hair follicles, they just create shorter, lighter hair that is barely noticeable. Women also get thinner hair or suffer from alopecia as they age but we do not generally notice because they cover up with appropriate hair pieces. There are also medical conditions and treatments that lead to thinner, patchy, or complete hair loss. None of the above should be a reason not to continue enjoying feminization activities.

If you are a Tgirl or in transition you may think that the above does not apply to you. Sadly, it is likely that the above will become relevant. When you take hormones what you get in softer features can be paid for elsewhere. Male baldness is caused by a reduction in testosterone. Hormone replacement therapy actively blocks testosterone. Even if you avoid the male pattern you can still end up with hair thinning. Also, when you start your new girl life, wigs and extensions can be an option until your hair grows out. And, anyway, it is always fun to change things up with designer hair as a fashion accessory. So, all-in-all, knowing your options is worthwhile.

Natural or Faux

The first choice to make is whether to use you own hair or cover it with a hair piece. Although people often associate wigs with crossdressing nowadays it is more acceptable for men to have longer hair as a natural style. This means you can grow out your hair a little and wear it in a ponytail, man bun, or top knot or other male style for work and such but have enough material to style it when you want a girl look. Alternatively, you may want to keep a reasonable male cut similar in length and body to a short haired female so you can again style your hair like them or use extensions to give it more body and length. If your feminization is a secret, you may prefer a traditional male cut and use a wig to totally transform when it comes to girl time. Below we will consider all the options so you can make a sensible choice.

Hair pieces are also great fashion accessories to change up your look. There is no reason to be stuck with your own natural hair colour. You can be a blonde, redhead, or brunette whatever your mood. You can have a range of short or long hair pieces some pre-styled and others that you can spend girl time styling yourself. If you visit a stylist or opt for a real makeover experience you can use their hair pieces or have them style your own. Some may fit you for a wig that you can purchase and take home. There are also a range of exotic hair pieces designed for more bizarre looks such as cosplay characters, metallics, and pastel colours. Once you understand the world of hair styling your choices for feminization are limitless.

Wigs, Extensions, and Weaves

The basic difference between a wig and an extension is the coverage. A wig covers the whole scalp whereas an extension covers only a part. A wig is easy to put on and take off because it is like a cap with the hair attached. A normal extension consists of additional human or synthetic hair that is dyed to match your own colour and is clipped, glued, or taped into your existing hair. A weave is a kind of extension sewn down into a braid of your own hair using the false strands. If you have a short girl style haircut, you can easily add length and volume with an extension or weave.

Extensions can come in a variety of forms from ponytails, to buns, to extra bangs or curls. And, for occasional purposes clip-in or tape ones are better because they can be easily removed. A weave or glue-in approach is intended to be worn for longer periods like days or weeks and should be done by a professional hairstylist for the best look. This is an option if you feminize more regularly or are in transition. The advantage of the latter is that they are fixed to your own hair and so more secure. A full wig is convenient but is less secure. It is just a cap and can move or slip off depending on your activity. Something to think about if you like to get passionate in the bedroom or do sports.

Wig Construction

Another thing to consider is the how realistic the hair looks and feels. There are many types of full wigs on the market from the fun inexpensive ones to more classy and expensive natural hair ones. An important factor here is how or to what degree you can style the hair.

First is whether your wig is made of human hair, animal hair, or synthetic. Human hair wigs have the most natural feel and movement. They can be treated almost the same as your own hair when it comes to styling and so on. Most human hair pieces use Asian hair which has a straight quality and can be dyed and styled for different hair pieces. European hair is the rarest. Animal hair has similar qualities to human hair but can feel coarse. The wig will tend to be cheaper though because the fibres can be obtained in greater volumes. Sometimes a mix of human and animal hair is used.

If you are on a budget synthetic hair is probably the cheapest. It has similar properties to human hair but is more sensitive to styling (in particular, heat treatments such as washing, drying, curling with tongs etc). Synthetic fibres also tend to have 'memory'. Once styled they retain some of the shape. Consequently, most synthetic wigs come pre-styled. You will need different ones to change your look. A more expensive human hair wig will be more versatile. So, if you are an occasional dresser then using a pre-styled piece will be quick and convenient. If you are a more regular girl then a natural wig might be a good option because it becomes part of your femme persona.

The way the wig is constructed also contributes to the cost. The usual approach is to attach the hair fibres to a cap which you then wear but the way this cap is constructed varies.

A wefted (or capless) wig: uses a loose framework of material a bit like a string bag. The strings or wefts are where the hair is attached to create layers. Usually the wefts are placed closer together at the crown to give more coverage and layering. These wigs are sometimes referred to as capless wigs because there is no material between the wefts. This can be helpful in that it allows your scalp to breathe so you don't get too hot or sweaty. But, it is also a limits what you can do with styling and the activities you can pursue because when you move the hair shifts and the wefts can become visible between the layers. If you are going to be a demure little creature who sits nicely or intend to use them for work or general situations, they should be okay. But if you are going to toss your hair, party, or do sports then you might want to think again.

Monofilament wigs: use a fuller cap of a more detailed net like material. In this case the individual strands of hair are sewn/tied through the net so that you get a much more natural coverage of the scalp. This overcomes the above limitations allowing you to style your hair more fully and gives the hair a more natural flow when you move around. A double monofilament wig works in the same way except that there are two layers of netting. The hairs are knotted (or sewn) into the first layer and then backed with a second layer making it more comfortable to wear. If your scalp is sensitive or you have thin hair or large bald areas this is a thing to consider because you are more likely to feel the knots against your skin. The downside is that the full cap covers all the scalp so they can be hotter to wear. Although, the material can be very lightweight because the netting is thin or sheer.

Lace front wigs: are similar to the above except they have an additional attachment of fine lace weave on the front. This allows additional hair to be sewn into the front piece to give a more natural looking hair line where the wig meets the face. If you want to style your hair off your face, for example in a side swept manner, these extra bits will make your wig almost undetectable. Likewise, If you have a receding hair line or that characteristic male M shape then these types of wigs will also be good because the edge of the wig will not be easily seen and you can shape your hairline into a nice female one. The same idea of lacing can also be used on the crown of the wig to give the hair a natural swirl. In this case if your hair style makes a feature of your crown or you need a parting to gather hair for an updo or bunches the wig will look more realistic.

Hand tied or machined: how the wig is manufactured is also important. With a machined wig the hairs or fibres are machine sewn into the weft so they can be produced quickly. In a hand-tied wig each strand of hair is sewn in place by a craftsman who can take upwards of three days to complete a single hair piece. This means that the hair appears and moves more naturally because a skilled wig maker can mimic how your hair would grow when they tie the hairs. Do not confuse hand tied with human hair, though. Both natural hair and synthetic fibres can be hand-tied. And, sometimes automatic stitching is finished and styled with some additional hand sewing to give them a more natural look.

Adjustable straps: a fashion or party wig often comes in one size only and can be loose or tight depending on the fit. A quality wig has adjustable strings or straps built into the cap which can be tightened to give a secure fit into the nape (or back of your head where it meets the neck). The strings can be tightened by up to an inch or more. This will make the wig hug the contours of your skull and be much more comfortable and secure to wear. Knowing that your hair piece is not going to come off easily or get skewed and give you away will do wonders to boost your girl confidence.

To summarize then, a hand-tied wig is seen as the most comfortable wig because the distribution of the hair makes it more natural and the density of the fibres makes it lighter to wear. If it is also a monofilament design, you won't feel the strap lines of the weft hugging your scalp. And with a double monofilament even the knots of the tied hair will be softened. With a lace front your hair will look as though it is really part of you. A play wig by comparison might have a much heavier cap which is machined more like a rug than a wig! So, if you want to feel more naturally feminine as opposed to playing dress up think about investing in some quality hair pieces with these features.

How to wear a wig

A lot of girls just wear their wig straight over their own hair but a little preparation will make things more comfortable and secure. Here is a four-step process to get your wig to fit properly:

Step 1 *prep your own hair*: if you have fuller hair then you will need to tame it a little with some bobby pins (or Kirby grips). Comb your hair and pin the longer strands flat against your scalp at the back. Likewise pin any fringe back to stop it flopping forward. If your hair is longer then tie it up in a couple of braids and wrap them behind your head and pin into the nape. All this flattens your existing hair back against your skull for a better fit.

Step 2 *put on a wig liner*: just to be confusing these are sometimes called wig caps and look a bit like stocking or tights material. They help hold your own hair in place and grip your wig to stop it slipping. Plus, it will help prevent sweat and skin oils getting onto your wig cap proper. Some liners come with elasticated bands that also help grip your head and the wig for a more secure fit. Obviously make sure the liner and band go behind your ears. Sounds obvious but you would be surprised how often people forget this, especially newbies.

Step 3 *put on the wig*: hold the wig out in front of you with the front facing away and the back towards you. Grip the top front portion of the wig (where the lace front might be) and dip your head forward towards it. Hold the front of the wig onto your forehead then flip the whole thing (and your head) backwards to pull the cap on. This way you can flick any longer hairs over your head and prevent them from getting in the way or being caught under the cap. Adjust the wig until it sits properly on your head. If it feels loose take it off and tighten the straps and repeat the process until you are happy with the fit.

Step 4 *adjust and pin*: If you need to secure the wig to your own hair and liner with some more bobby pins. Consider whether you need pins either side of the forehead, just above the ears, and just behind the ears or nape. With a wefted wig put the pin through the gap in the weft and into your own hair. For a fuller cap wig pin the edges of the wig under the hair line to the liner. If it still feels wobbly, and it shouldn't by now, or if you prefer, use some double-sided tape. Stick a strip inside the wig cap and then it will stick to the wig liner when you pull the wig on. The wig can be a bit more difficult to adjust though.

Okay, that is your wig on. If it is pre-styled you can move on to accessories. And if not, you will need to style your hair. We will get to that in the next chapter. For now, just arrange the hair around your face and get it to hang nicely and enjoy the vision of the girly you. You might also want to comb it out a little. Such a femme thing to just sit and comb your hair wistfully in front of the mirror. Girls with extra long hair need to comb out every night to prevent tangles and knots. One hundred strokes of the comb before bedtime is often a mother's advice. A staple of romantic fiction has bedtime grooming as the point in the plot when sisters swap stories and secrets while one brushes the hair of the other. Anyhow, you will need to learn to care for your new hair and combing is an essential.

Care and maintenance

Before we move on it is worth taking a few moments on how to look after your hair pieces so that they stay in good condition and last. Obviously, false hair is not going to grow so it will get worn the more you wear it. Also, it will get dirty just like normal hair. And, if you damage it then not much can be done except to re-style with a cut so hopefully the following tips will be useful.

The first thing to note is the difference between human hair and synthetic fibres. Both do not like too much heat but the latter can melt. A heat resistant synthetic wig may take temperatures up to 350°F/180°C. So, it is good practice to let your wigs dry naturally rather than using a hair dryer. Likewise, if you apply tongs and curlers which are too hot you will spoil the hair. A bit of styling like this is not out of the question just be careful to use the lower settings. If in doubt refer to the instructions that come with the piece.

Never shower with your wig on. This sounds like a super femme thing to do and the ideal way to clean it but it will knot and tangle just like real hair. Plus, the heat in the water may make it frizz – yes wigs frizz too! The ideal cleaning procedure is to soak with shampoo and conditioner in cold water. If you wash it and rub like regular hair it will tangle. Comb out the shampoo and conditioner as much as you can and then rinse with warm water. If there are tangles then comb these out as well. Then hang the wig and let it dry naturally. There are special products for hair pieces that have milder chemicals than you apply to normal hair and there are also special wig combs that help with detangling.

Store the hair piece using a mannequin head or a wig hook which is like a normal hook but larger and shaped to give the hair form. Hanging the wig also allows the strands to hang properly so you will minimise the tangles and kinking. Remember that synthetic hairs have a little memory so they will take on the storage shape. So, don't just stuff it in the draw! If the wig is only used occasionally then add a cover to protect it from accumulating dust and other particles.

And, finally on this. You may want to sleep in your wig. That though is a bad idea. As your head moves and you squiggle it will just knot up and get tangled. Okay if you are prepared to put in the effort to smooth it out. But if it is synthetic then you might find that a bad hair day turns into a permanent look because as we have already said synthetic fibres have memory.

Extensions with shorter hair

If you have enough hair, extensions are easier to wear by a mile. They are attached directly to your hair so feel more natural and are difficult to dislodge. Plus, there is no need to faff with a liner and so forth. The secret though is to choose extensions that are not too long and that mix naturally with your shorter hair. Aim for 16-18 inches (30-40 cms) or less – that is just over a foot to a foot and half. This will give you hair lengths from level with the chin to just below the shoulder. If you want shorter ones than that, you can cut them to size quite easily. Longer ones will be heavier and pull on your scalp and hair.

An extension is composed of a single length of weft (like a wig) with the hair attached. When you choose your wefts get enough pieces for the volume you want. Also check the thickness or thinness of the extension to make sure it matches well with your own hair. One or two extensions are usually enough but get more if you want to experiment. If you use too many, they will pull your hair, can droop, and may expose the clips or tape so lighter is better. Match your hair colour as closely as you can. Human hair extensions can be dyed just like normal hair.

Here is a little procedure to fix your extensions in place:

Step 1 *prep the hair*: obviously, you don't want to have greasy or oily hair, so that the clips (or tape) will hold, and the dirt will not rub off on the extension. Wash and condition your hair as you would normally. We are not going to go through a hair care routine here but if you are using your own hair add hair nourishment and care to your regular pamper sessions.

Step 2 *separate*: the extension is going to fit between two separate layers of your hair so that the clips (or whatever) are hidden. Decide where you want to place the extension in relation to the top of your head. Gather all the hair above this line and secure with a hair tie or a clip. This will be more or less challenging depending on the length of your hair and how close to the crown you are.

Step 3 *tease*: now you have two sections of hair. The gathered part is one layer and the rest of your hair is the second layer. Tease the edge of the second layer where it joins the scalp to get it ready for clipping or taping. That is, use a comb or your fingers and just ruffle the hairs up a bit and then smooth out.

Step 4 *attach*: take the extension and position it over the second layer as close to the top of the hair (and scalp) as you can and then attach it to your own hair. If you have more than one extension apply them similarly. Adjust and redo until you are happy with the positioning. Now unfasten your top layer and let the hair fall (arrange itself) over the new extension.

That's it, now you have longer girl hair. Success with this depends on how much hair you have to work with. Remember that short-girl hair often has quite a lot of volume compared to male hair and may well cover the ears and extend to the chin. If you are struggling with the extension or it looks too obvious, can you grow your hair out a bit to make that first layer? If you have the same sort of volume and length as a Mop-top (that famous Paul McCartney *Beatles* haircut, where he tossed his hair on video) or something similar you probably have enough for extensions.

Another alternative is a Halo extension. In this form you get a virtually full head of hair attached to a circular band. The band fits around your head under the first layer of hair and can be pinned under a fringe area at the front. Yet another variation is to give your hair more volume at the back by bunching up your own hair to make a small bun. The extension then lays over the bun giving the appearance of more contour and hair volume. You can also gather your hair at the back and clip on a ponytail if that is your look. There are many variations to these ideas. The main point of extensions though is that they give you a natural look and are not that difficult to apply. The more elaborate you need to be the more you should be thinking about going to a full wig. Remember all that stuff weighs something and will start to pull and stretch your hair.

Looking after extensions

Do the same precautions for wigs apply for extensions? Well usually extensions are human hair, so they are tougher than synthetics and are also designed to stay in for longer. A weave for example might be in for 3-4 months. So, it is not difficult to figure out that you will have to wash and sleep wearing your extensions. Most of the maintenance advice for wigs still applies but there are some caveats.

You should brush your extensions daily to stop them getting tangled at the base or the clip area but do it gently. Avoid tugging the hair as this will just pull at the clips or other attachments and weaken the hold of the hair in the weft. Don't use too much heat in the shower and use milder (recommended) products on your head. When you wash your hair with the extensions in place only shampoo the top layer and leave the conditioner for the second layer (mid to and ends of your hair). Make sure you stand upright so that the water runs down your hair and onto your back this will minimise tangling and knotting.

Never go to bed with your extensions wet or even semi dry this just encourages tangling and matting which will make it more difficult to comb. So, no flopping on the bed and falling asleep or anything else after a shower. Take the time to hand comb your extensions until they are dry. Wear some lingerie to make it a fun and intimate girl moment.

Alternatively, watch a movie while your hair dries. It is also a good idea to secure your hair with something like a hair net to avoid tangles and your partner pulling on the clips and attachments if they trap the strands while you are sleeping.

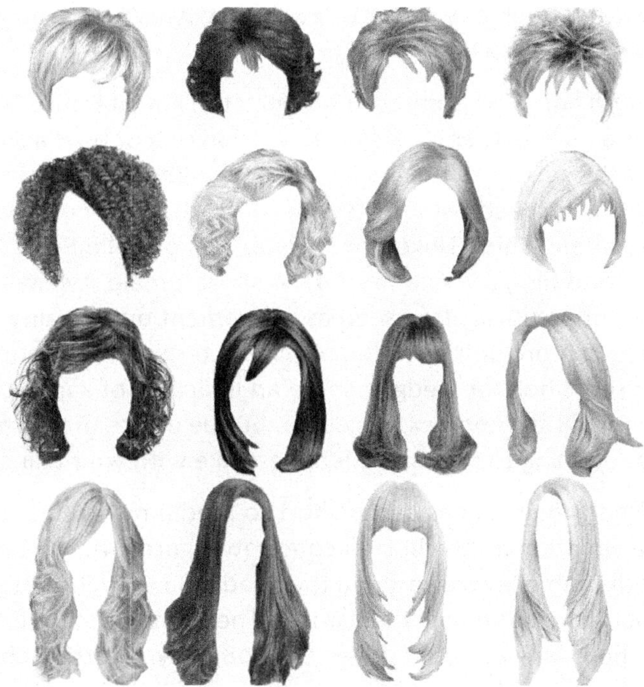

Figure 14 Various hair styles (ear, chin, shoulder, and armpit length)

A hair net designed for everyday use (not just at bedtime) is called a snood and can look super feminine with pinned up hair or just to gather your longer tresses off your face and shoulders. Check out some 1940s styles to get the look. If you do sports like horse riding or where you need to wear a helmet or hard hat this sort of arrangement can be more convenient than pinning up your hair.

Hair Length and texture

Women have a wonderfully diverse range of hair styles so before we get into choosing your own style it might be worth defining at a few general hair terms. This will also stand you in good order if you want to search for a pre-styled wig and do not know what to look for.

First up is hair length. A short male haircut would be a buzz cut or a crew cut close to the scalp, but a long cut would not go much past the ears. A short style with more volume is often called an ivy league because it is popular with preppy college guys. Women in contrast have a choice of five main lengths.

Ear length hair is considered very short (top line of Figure 14) with styles such as a pixie cut, or back shaved version of a bob, or a side shave but usually the rest of the hair such as the fringe is kept longer. These are difficult to succeed with unless your face is already elf-like or a classic female shape. Think Tinkerbell in *Peter Pan* or Halle Berry as Jinx in the James Bond film, *Die Another Day*. A short female style with shaving or severe undercuts is often seen as a comment on sexuality. A butch cut indicates a more dominant female character whereas a softer pixie cut, a very short bob, or wedge can be an indicator of sapphic tendencies. These are all stereotypes, of course, but be aware of the messages you may be sending to males and females alike with your hair style.

Chin length hair is considered short to medium with the most obvious style a variation on the bob (second row Figure 14). In a bob the hair is cut at the same level all around the head at jaw level. That is well above the shoulders but below the ear tips. There are many variations such as blunt bob, angled bob, inverted bob, asymmetrical bob etc etc. Examples, Uma Thurman in *Pulp Fiction*, and Julia Roberts' street hair in *Pretty Woman*. Because of its boy style it was once seen as a daring cut by Flappers and women's right activists but now it is a common place softer female cut.

Shoulder length hair is considered medium and one of the most popular choices (row three in Figure 14). The hair can be styled in many ways but usually the main variation is the degree of layering and feathering. In layering the hair towards the crown is cut shorter than the longer hair underneath. This gives the layered effect and different volume qualities which help frame the face. Feathering refers to how the ends of the hair are cut to give the hair different textures. The look varies depending on the degree of straightness, waviness, or curl of the hair. A long bob (or lob) is a popular choice that can curve in towards the face under the jawline. Side partings, a shag, or messy look are also popular but there are lots of freer styles.

A shag cut is layered and feathered on the top and sides like in row one of Figure 14 but can also be used for longer hair. Check out Jane Fonda who is famous for many stylish looks from soft curls through to the more edgy shag with blunt bangs and angled jaw in the 1971 film *Klute* (her first Oscar winning role). Other good examples for this category are Michelle Pfeiffer in *Scarface*, the iconic Farrah Fawcett or Cheryl Ladd in the original *Charlie's Angels TV series,* Jennifer Aniston's, 'Rachel' look. from hit comedy *Friends*, and Sharon Stone in the movie *Total Recall.*

Chest (or Armpit) length is considered long (row four of Figure 14). A characteristic of this style is that it touches your shoulder blades at the back and can just cover or lie on your boobs at the front. This suits long straight, curly or wavy hairstyles and can be layered, feathered, balayaged (where swatches of hair are hand painted differently to your main colour), a longer shag or messy which is often referred to as surfer girl – think Baywatch. The back can be tapered or cut square. A soft layered style can produce a sweet look while more wave is princess and curly gives a lusty and pre-Raphaelite look. Think Debra Messing with those lovely copper curls in *Wedding Date*, Jacqueline Bisset's iconic 1960s look, and Amy Adams in *Enchanted.*

Midback to tailbone is considered very long. Normally the hair tapers to a point and can be anything from pin straight through thick waves to extremely curly. The weight of the hair means that if it is not in an 'up do', pinned, braided or bunched then the options of styling are limited. Free long straight hair with a square front fringe is typical of the Hime look in Japanese Manga/Anime. More curly is Lady Godiva or Mermaid. Think Julia Roberts in *Pretty Woman* (without the bob wig), Jane Seymour, as Solitaire, in *Live and Let Die*, Brooke Shields in *Blue Lagoon,* and Katherine Ross in *Butch Cassidy and the Sundance Kid*.

Another distinctive quality of hair is texture or thickness. Hair can be silky smooth, straight, wavy, curly, or tightly curled. Each one can make you look quite different and can frame your face in unique ways. To change from straight to curly or curly to straight you are going to need some tools. Most typically these involve heat to change the hold of the hair fibres. To straighten you will need hair tongs. To curl you will need a curling iron or rollers. A decent hairdryer is also a must with head attachments for blow drying your hair in various ways. Blow dried hair with volume created by air in between or under the fibres is called a blow-out. A diffuser attachment is a must for naturally curly hair because it helps spread the heat and so dries all the curls evenly and to the same tightness. You can style a human hair wig with these tools but because synthetic wigs are more sensitive to heat it is better to buy the wig with the right hair texture in the first place.

Longer hair is also more prone to splitting. Split (or dead) ends make the hair look more feather like and can knot or tangle. They occur when the hair gets dry and brittle and frays like the ends of a rope. This happens when you use heat on your hair to straighten, curl, or blow dry but they can also occur from chemical damage such as dyes and strong cleaning products. You will need to comb the hair more often and ensure you use gentle shampoo and conditioners to nourish the hair properly. Sometimes the only solution is a cut and style. So, if you have a worn hairpiece don't just bin it. Take it to a hair stylist for a professional cut and shape. Yes, it will be shorter and maybe not your ideal look, but you will still get some more hours of enjoyment out of it.

Basic Hair Terms

After length and texture, it is useful to know some other terms so that you can look at hair styles in magazines or online and understand how they are constructed. When you start to gain this insider knowledge you will appreciate the artistry and beauty of female hair. For convenience, the basic approaches can be grouped into the following features and attributes.

Fringe: another way to differentiate hair styles is by how the hair falls over the front hairline onto the forehead. The technical term for the locks of hair that covers this area down to the eyebrows are bangs. The most popular style is to cut them straight although they can be ragged or ruffled or combed or in a U shape. The bangs might also be curled like a comma (or kiss curl). When the hair is parted in the centre the bangs fall either side framing the face. These can be straight or curled or tighter ringlets. When the parting is to the left or right the bangs can be swept to one side which looks super sexy especially with a longer style that covers one eye. Tucking the fringe hair over the ears can also look extra cute. Pinning it off the face not only looks pretty but is practical as well. Audrey Hepburn was famous for a pinned style of hair with shorter bangs. The Bettie Page look with straight bangs and silky shoulder length hair is popular with crossdressers but exceedingly difficult to carry off. The reason being that the longer angular bangs show up the brow ridge and make the face appear more mannish. A parting and swept or wavy look is often better, for example the burlesque star and model, Dita Von Teese.

Bouffant: when the bangs are styled upwards off the face and combed back you get a Bouffant look made famous by the likes of Jackie Kennedy. This style was popular in Victorian times and was revived by Bridget Bardot and Raquel Welch in the later nineteen fifties with the half up do and sex kitten look. When the rest of the hair is pulled up into an Up-Do on top of the head you get the Amy Whitehouse Beehive effect which can be given variety by arranging the bangs. An alternative is called *Le Pouf* with a lower pull back or less volume. Think early Jessica Alba or Nicole "snooki" Polizzi (aka Jersey shore).

Bunched: when a section of hair is gathered it is referred to as bunched. When all the hair is gathered and tied in a single bunch it makes a ponytail. It is still called a ponytail even if the point of bunching is to the side or top of the head not just the back. When the hair is collected into two bunches the proper name is twin tails. If the two bunches are long and to the sides they are referred to as doggy ears. Although, if the hair is also braided, they are referred to as pigtails. Technically though, free (not braided) short hair bunches either side of the top or bottom of the side or back of the head are what is meant by pigtails. A variation of the twin tale style in which the hair is first wrapped into a bun before falling into the tail is referred to as Odango. The latter is super cute and appears a lot in Anime and Cosplay. The bunches can be secured with an elasticated hair tie and accessorised in various ways.

Braids: refer to a length of hair that is usually divided into three sections that are crossed over one another (or plaited) to create a pattern. There are many many types of braids all which give different looks. The main point is to tame longer voluminous hair and pin it up, so it doesn't get in the way. Here are a few common approaches:

Simple (or basic): is probably the first hair style girls with long hair learn. The hair is separated into three bunches and then plaited to the ends and secured with a hair tie. The look can be different depending on how tight or loose the plaits are and the volume of the hair. This style is the one used with pony or pigtails.

Fishtail braids combine a regular ponytail with a braid. In this case the bottom part of the ponytail is tied off and then separated into two groups which are then braided separately and joined back together. The latter is easier to reach and do for a beginner.

French Braid (or Oklahoma) is a classy work look. The hair is gathered from between the temples and split into three strands. As the plait works downwards from the crown to nape extra hair is brought in from the sides. At the end it becomes a ponytail and is tied off. This gives a nice tight pattern on the back and into the sides of the head. It is a popular look for gymnasts and sporty girls. And also the staple of the farm girl or homesteader wife look.

Dutch Braids are the same as the French Braids except that the hair is wrapped under rather than over during the plaiting. This makes the braid stand out more on the back of the head. A variation of both of these types is the reverse braid which starts at the nape and works upwards to the crown. The excess material is then tied off and styled into a bun or topknot. Revealing the wispy (or baby) hair at the nape of the neck in this way can be highly sensual.

Waterfall braids are like French braids that start at the temple and go across the side of the head to the back. When some of the plaiting is left free to hang it gives the waterfall effect. These can look very neat and sweet. And are popular with younger girls. You will see a lot of female athletes with these types of braids.

Crown (or halo) braids are braids that wrap around the top of the head. First the hair is divided down the middle of the back of the head. Then a French or Dutch braid is created on one side working up towards the forehead. The second side is then braided in the same way starting at the forehead and working towards the back. The two braids are then arranged and pinned together to make an oval or halo shape. This is a popular bride look with the veil pinned into or under the braid.

Milkmaid braids use two pigtail braids. The braiding starts lower than other braids at the side of the head or by the ears. Each braid is then lifted over the top of the head and pinned. As a variant and if the hair is longer the braids can be looped or gathered in various ways. Ideally the hair is parted down the back to make the bunches and to give a very neat line up the back of the head. If the braids are left to hang by the ears, they create a looser and more shield-maiden (or Viking) style.

Corn row braids are tighter sequences of braids that run over the head and leave some of the scalp visible. They are popular with men, women, and children from non-Caucasian ethnic groups and can be styled in various ways. They don't really suit the crossdresser because the overall appearance is a very short. We mention them here only because a corn row braid can be used as a weft for more permanent hair extensions if you are a 24/7 girl.

There are lots of other variations too *such as Box braids (*popular with African Americans*)* and *Rope braids.* The latter uses just two bunches of hair which are twisted as they are plaited so they look like a thick rope. This is a nice loose style and works for longer hair with lots of volume. Think Rapunzel. You can also braid using more than three gathers of hair. And, of course, braids can be accessorised by working ribbons of different colours into the plait which is very soft and feminine. You see this a lot in gymnastics or dance.

<u>Twists and Wraps:</u> involve gathering the hair in some way to perform various twists and then pinning it in place. Below are some common types.

Buns: The classic example of a twist is a bun. To make a bun you first gather your hair into a ponytail and secure with hair ties at the end and at the bottom of the hair close to the head. Now twist (or wrap and coil the) hair around the base and pin in place. Simple and classy and the staple Ballerina look. The bun can appear on top or back of the head or at the base of the neck. Sometimes a braid (such as fish tail) is used to give more pattern and texture. There are so many ways to do this that it is impossible to mention them all.

Double Bun (or Fallera): uses two buns usually one either side of the head and was first popular in Valencia as part of the Fallas festival. So, this suits darker hair with a Spanish feel or complexion. The other name for it is the Princess Leia (from *Star Wars*). When the buns are smaller and towards the back with longer tails, they become Odango. Rei in the more recent Star Wars movies has a triple bun look worked into a ponytail.

Doughnut Bun: for this you need a donut accessory. Make a ponytail as in the previous single bun method. Slip the ponytail through the hole in the donut and slide it up to your head. Now wrap the rest of the ponytail around to hide the donut until there is none left adjusting for a tight fit and then pinning to secure. This suits a prim efficient secretary or librarian look especially with glasses.

Loose (or half) Bun: is used for a casual or messy hair look. This is like the full bun except that you don't tie off the base. Gather up a section of your hair at the back and make a quick ponytail. Wrap the hair around the base until you have gone all the way around at least once and secure. Now just arrange as you want. Probably the first time you do a bun it will look like this. If it is too neat just tease out the hair a bit to make it messy. This has a sensual look between prim and softer which can be ultra-sexy.

Chignons: are like buns except that they appear at the nape of the neck. Separate out your hair close to the nape to get two bunches straighten them out like ponytails. Now tie the two ponytails loosely together. Wrap in any excess hair and pin in place. Now adjust to get the look you want by teasing the hair. Again, there are lots of variations on this with different patterns and textures. We will look at two variations called topsy-tail and stick hair that are easy for beginners in the next chapter. These are nice sophisticated looks suited to the lady boss or a softer confident mature look.

French twist: this is a very elegant style and again comes in all kinds of varieties. A simple twist is as follows. Sweep all your hair to one side at the back. Keep a hold of the hair and then pin up the middle of the back of the head with bobby pins to stop the hair falling back into position. Hold the gathered hair underneath and comb for a smooth look. Next twist the hair in the opposite direction to the way you swept the hair (lifting or) pulling upwards as you do so. Twist until you have a nice tension and then roll and tuck the excess hair under and pin in place. Tidy away any loose ends into the top of the twist for a neat look or leave for a loose look. If you find it difficult to secure you can always use a hair comb or clip to hold it in place. This is a very chic look ideal for formal events or work. Jeri Ryan (aka 7 of 9), in the TV series, *Star Trek Voyag*er, has a mind-blowingly sexy French twist thing going on.

Up Dos: involve arranging the hair so that the strands runs upwards rather than downwards. This style has two purposes first is to lift the hair off the shoulders and nape of the neck. The second purpose is to take the weight of longer hair by attaching the ends to the head. This also keeps it nicely out of the way. So with these criteria we can see that some buns and braids are also simple forms of Up Do. However, Up Do's are usually much more elaborate using a mixture of techniques to give a very neat or refined appearance.

We mentioned the Bouffant and Beehive which are modern Up Dos but there are also some timeless classics. How the hair is arranged at the sides or parted make all the difference. We won't go through all these because they need a stylist or help to complete but some popular styles were bonnet hair with ringlet bangs and side buns (think Jane Austen), Barley curls (waves or ringlet curves without bangs and flat to the sides of the head aka Agatha Christie dramas), and Gibson girl (where the hair is piled high and loose at the sides and folded into a bun on top of the head, aka Jane Seymour in the film *Somewhere in time*).

Nowadays, unless your hair is exceptionally long and unmanageable an Up Do is left for formal occasions like weddings or proms, a formal dance or visit to the theatre. If you want to see some stunningly beautiful examples search online for Bridal hair. When matched with naked shoulders and upper chest (or décolletage) they present a very elegant almost princess look. Gathering and pulling all the hair upwards to pile it on top and secure with a bun or topknot is a typical Victorian and Edwardian look (18th-19th century). Exposing the wispy hair at the nape and the area behind the ears is also very sensual especially if this softness is contrasted with some neat lines like the parting for bunches or tighter curls like ringlets or braided patterns.

Hair Accessories

So far, we have talked about basic hair looks but there is a lot we can do to pretty-things up even more or make knock-out statements by using hair accessories. The things you need can be divided into the following groups:

Combs: the function of a comb is to keep the hair strands neat and untangled. Everyone understands the idea of a *wide toothed comb* which easily detangles hair but there are many different types of comb for female hair. The wide toothed variety normally comes as a paddle style. A *fine-toothed comb* is flat and has narrower more dense teeth to be used after the wide toothed comb to get the strands to lay properly. This can be used to pry knots loose gently without snagging or pulling the hair out and is more like a man-comb. A *rat tail comb* is used to get very straight partings – the rat tail part is used to separate the hair and the comb part to brush out the sides of the parting. A *pin tail comb* is used for more delicate and intricate work in styling. They are used to pick up strands of hairs and gather or to attach to rollers for curl. And last, a *teasing comb* has smaller denser bristles to help remove knots but also to fluff up thinner hair so that it can be given more body for styling.

Pins: we have met the ubiquitous *Bobby pin* (or Kirby grip) already, this is the oldest and most used type of pin and comes in a U shape with a flat side and corrugated side to grip the hair. There are many other types of pin. *Barrette pins* are wider and flatter with a tension flap in the centre which can gather swatches of hair. They can come in all sorts of designs and the wider end can be decorated with patterns like flowers or swirls. *Hair stick pins* look like pencils or chopsticks and are used to hold a bun without normal pins or ties. A variant is a wooden pin that can be carved in a variety of ways for natural earthy look. *Spiral pins* are used like bobby pins but to control more curly hair. Long *decorative pins* come in a variety of shapes and have a longer pin part and the top of the U shape has some detail like flowers, butterflies, or pearls designed to be visible or 'float' on the hair.

Slides and cuffs: a comb pin is referred to as a slide. Normally they are semi-circular with pin shaped teeth to grip the hair. They can be metal, plastic, or wooden and the top of the comb (or arch) can be plain or decorated. The teeth or comb part usually keep the slide in place and can be narrow or wide. A cuff can also give you an interesting look by making your ponytail stand up more from the head. They can be cylindrical, or cone shaped, with different lengths for added lift and made of all sorts of materials and colours from metallic to decorative.

<u>Clips:</u> have a hinge and fastening to hold the hair. The pin side slides into the hair and the top part clips to it leaving the surface visible so they can be decorated in various ways. A *banana clip* consists of two combs (or slides) with a hinge at one end and catch at the other. Hair is gathered between the combs and the clip fastened. This helps with vertical bunching to secure twists and is often used for short to medium hair instead of a bun. The *snap clip* is like a barrette pin except the central part is in tension so that it flips closed when pressed to grab the hair. Snaps are often used by younger girls to hold the hair off the face and come in all sorts of colours. Adults can also use plainer ones for the same reason or to flatten an unruly lock of hair. *Crocodile clips* are long plain thin pins with jaws and teeth on the inside and a strong (sprung) hinge. These can help with holding a bun but are mainly used to hold hair temporarily out of the way while other parts of the hair are being styled and fixed. You might also use them to hold up the hair while you take a bath to avoid getting it wet.

<u>Grips:</u> are like clips in that they have a hinge but normally come with comb teeth and do not clip or lock. The hinge is usually tensioned with a spring. They act like hands to gather hair and then hold it. The *butterfly grip* is an example with two wings and the hinge in the middle. Just gather the hair and open the grip and then close it on the hair. Claw grips look like the jaws of a pickup digger or indeed a bird claw. They are more curved than butterfly clips and so can grab more hair. Grips can be used to hold hair up temporarily while you wash or bathe but also for a looser or messy hair look that can be very chic. They provide a quick way of putting your hair up while you are on the go.

<u>Bands:</u> a hair band is a strip of fabric or other material bent into a horseshoe shape and designed to grip the sides of the head and hold hair off the face. The *Alice band* is the typical example so called because it is worn by Alice in Wonderland. Sometimes the underside of the band

can have a small comb attachment for more grip. The band can be thinner or thicker, coloured or decorated, depending on the look you want. Simple ones are just straight plastic, but fabric and elasticated ones can give different patterns. Velvet and diamante ones are incredibly chic. And ones with cat ears are used for a cute look at parties. A band of some sort with flowers woven into the top is called a garland and when extended to the rest of the hair produces a sweet rustic look.

Tiaras: a tiara is a metal version of a band that slides into the top of the hair. The top can be shaped off the head with jewels and stones which is popular for the princess, prom queen, pageant, or the evening gown look. The idea is to show wealth and/or status and can be matched with necklaces and earrings. More elaborate elf style ones inspired by the *Lord of the Rings* franchise are popular for the fairy look. A mixture of all the above techniques is used to create Bridal hair where the band or tiara is also used to attach the veil.

Ties, Ribbons, and Bows: A *basic tie* is just an elastic circular band that can be slipped over and twisted around a gathering of hair to hold it firmly. For example, to hold a ponytail or the end of a braid. Normally the ties are low key but they can be embellished. The most obvious is to thread the tie through a little coloured ball or attach a bow. A looser tie with a fabric covering is called a scrunchy. These are worn at the base of a ponytail or bun. A small scrunchy with a silk or more fluffy texture is often added to the bun in the Odango style. For a looser look a girl will wear the scrunchy on her wrist and then quickly tie up the hair when she needs to control it or concentrate then take it out again when relaxing. This allows you to flip between more formal and casual styles.

Ribbons were the main way of securing pigtails and ponytails before elastic ties became available. Because of their sweet appeal they are still used by younger girls but also young female adults. They double to hide the basic tie and give some decoration. Ribbons can be long or short, wide or thin, and edged with lace or other decorations. Fabric varies from cloth to silk. Thinner ribbons are used for a plain look and can be woven into braids for a multicolour effect. The wider ones are used for a sweet cute look.

The appeal of a ribbon is that the easiest way to tie it off is in a bow. The shape and looping of the bow can give different looks. A wide ribbon bow around the base of a ponytail is a staple of rock-n-roll girls and also as a decorative flourish for gymnasts and cheerleaders. Thicker ribbons look super cute on doggy ears especially with bigger bows. Shorter smaller bows on pigtails can look very sweet and girl-next-door particularly when on the bottom of the head. The fifties housewife look can also use a ribbon to hold the hair off the face. A chic version is to use a scarf instead of a ribbon. And, when a scarf or handkerchief is used more like a band and tied at the nape it has a peasant girl or gypsy quality.

Because bows have such a pretty female quality the actual bow part of the ribbon is now often sold separately and pre-made as a decorative finish to clips and slides. This style is often used by older or more mature women. A larger silk bow might be used with a hair slide to help hide the pin or clip of a bun. A decorative pin might be finished with a bow so it floats on the hair. A bow may also disguise the visible part of the hinge or be used to give a plain hair style a boost. Other decorative fixes include butterflies and flowers. So plenty of choice.

Hair and your inner girl

Just in case you are thinking these are all very pretty but what have they got to do with feminization when all we can do is wear a hair piece? Don't miss out on this ultimate girly experience. Learning to braid, bun, or bunch your hair is an essential element of your socialisation as female. All girls learn to do it. Even a loose or haphazard look can be cute or sensual depending on how it is done. And choosing accessories and combos will give you hours of girly fun.

How you choose to wear your hair is a great way to express your inner girl. A medium to long human hair wig can be styled in just about the same ways as genuine hair. And all of the above, apart from say extra curl, only require pinning, tying, twisting or clipping so don't need heat at all. You can also use a little hair spray to give some hold but not too much and always wash it out after you use your hair piece. And, if you like one of the above looks but do not want to style it yourself you can buy pre-styled wigs and accessorize. There are many wigs available with buns and braids, twists, chignons and so on built in. These are sometimes referred to as hair systems rather than just wigs.

If you are being feminized your mistress or partner might want a certain look. Doggy ears, pigtails, and odango with elaborate ribbons is a go to look for sissy girls. Ringlets, braids, up dos and so forth go with those little party and quince dresses. Milkmaid braids and a tight neat look are good for, you guessed it, Maids. In feminization training the emphasis is on treating you like a girl not necessarily to hide all your man features. Making it obvious that you are a feminized man is part of the appeal and there is no way to do that better than doing your hair and accessorising girl style. In contrast, if the objective is to be as authentic as possible these techniques and styles will make you more passable. So, whether you are a 24/7 girl or just a social dresser, there are lots of reasons why you might be interested in learning one or more of the above.

Finally, on this, one thing that every girl should experience is that special day. If you haven't dreamed or thought about it already, consider booking a bridal makeover appointment. Not only will you get to wear lovely lingerie but also a gorgeous dress and have your hair pinned and braided in a bridal style. If you have a group of 'girl' friends, consider doing bridesmaids as well and pose for some pictures. And, if you think you are too old for all that it can be understated or you can turn yourself out as mother-of-the-bride which is another whole look with more mature but special hair styles too. Who knows perhaps one day you will experience all that for real! If that is not for you, consider having a Quinceanera style party just to celebrate your transition from male to female. Or go chic with posh frocks, hats, and fancy fascinators for a day out sipping champagne at the races.

Shopping List

Okay lots of ideas and new things to consider. Let's put together another shopping list.

First up is your hair pieces. To start you probably need just one but which one? A synthetic wig starts in the region of $/£50 for an out-of-the-box model which means it is pre-styled. If you know what you want and browse styles beforehand this can be a good first option. A human hair wig is £/$300-500 for a given length, colour, and basic cut which you can then style yourself. A bespoke wig specially designed for your own look can set you back £/$2000-3000. The price within each type varies depending on the cap details, lace front, and so on that we discussed earlier. A semi-custom wig will fall between the basic and bespoke wig costs. In this case you basically get a standard wig size, colour and shape but it can be altered to fit your requirements.

There are many on-line wig suppliers but do be careful because there are a few pirates out there. For extra safety check to see if they have the usual things like contact and customer service numbers. Crossdressing stores are generally reputable, but the choice will be limited mostly to synthetic and fashion wigs at affordable prices. A fashion (or celebrity) wig is one that is styled for a currently popular trend or fad. So, a choice if you want a pre-styled something that is of the moment. It is possible to spend a lot of money if you get wig-addicted and like lots of styles or buy different lengths or colours. Anyhow, if you have a local crossdressing store or a makeover provider that sells wigs and makeup it is worth booking an appointment. That way you can avoid internet risks and try on some pieces to find the one you like.

Wherever you decide to purchase your wig you will need some measurements. Wigs come in four basic sizes: Ultra Petite, Petite, Average and Large. Six measurements determine the size and fit: circumference (round from back to front, forehead to nape), front to back (forehead to nape), side to side over the forehead (from ear to ear), side to side over the top (like a hair band), temple to temple across the back, and the nape of the neck. An average size has the measurements: 22-22.5", 14-14.5", 12-12.5", 12.5-13", 14.5-15", and 5-5.5" for the above. An adjustable wig can give you an extra inch or less on the circumference. And remember that these sizes are designed for female heads so you might have slightly bigger measurements depending on your build. Another reason to go to a crossdressing store or wig shop to try them on.

If you prefer extensions, you can go to a salon or buy them on-line and fit yourself. Salon extensions can cost £/$150-700 per visit for a set that might last several months but it can go over £/$1000 depending on what you want length wise, the extension quality, or weight of hair. DIY clip in ones can cost you £/$100-200 but be careful what you buy because preferably you want the human hair ones not synthetics (which will always be cheaper). There are also double-sided tape ones too. On-line stores like amazon and ebay do synthetics from £/$10 upwards but make sure you count the number of pieces in the price because you may need several. A halo piece might be £/$30 upwards.

The best quality hair for both wigs and extensions is Remy hair. Remy is human hair that has been collected in a way that preserves the cuticle and to ensure the strands stay aligned. This means that the lay of the hair is smoother and they do not catch as much when you brush so are less likely to tangle. Remy hair is also virgin hair which refers to human hair that has never been treated with dyes or chemicals. The quality of the hair is softer to the touch and appears more natural than other types. All Remy hair is virgin but not all virgin hair is Remy. So, the basic, but not the only difference, is that non-Remy hair is collected from hairbrushes and floors of hair salons.

If you are on a budget, try not to skimp. Synthetic fibres of lower quality have more shine and may look false. Limit the number of wigs you buy rather than getting super cheap ones. If you are not sure about length read the next chapter to see how hair length helps to frame your face and add to its feminine qualities. But as a rough guide stick to the middle three lengths of chin, shoulder, and armpit-length. This will give you some flexibility in softening your male features without being too onerous to manage. The longer of these will give you options to style if they are not synthetic or pre-styled. Stick with one colour to start and buy more pieces as you get comfortable with wearing them and know more about what you want.

Most hair accessories can be bought quite cheaply (<£/$10 per item) on-line, in high street fashion stores, or pharmacies. Bobby pins and basic ties are ultra-cheap and come in sets of 20-30 for £/$3 or less. Stock up on those. They tend to go missing. Wig cap/liners are in the same price zone though a quality one might go up to £/$8. If you are a regular wig wearer, you will need a few so you can wash and re-cycle. A decent comb or set of combs come in at £/$10 for a paddle brush and less for pin tails and the like.

Mannequin heads for wig storage range from £/$2 to 20+ depending on how much detail you want on the head. A plain polystyrene one is all you need for shape but you can get them with neck, shoulders, and face detail for display purposes. Wig hooks that hang in a wardrobe and dust bags are <£/$10. You can also get portable wig cases that will fit in normal luggage and are good if you femme up when on business trips or vacation. Straighteners, curlers, and tongs all vary in price from £/$30 to hundreds depending on the quality, settings, and range of attachments.

As a starter accessory set get a multipack of bobby pins, some slides and grips, an Alice band or two, some elastic pony tail ties, a few scrunchies, ribbons (if you like them), and some decorative clips with bows and so on. This will allow you to try out a lot of the things discussed in this chapter. Then as your look develops buy more of what you like. Because these items are so cheap it is a good idea to browse when you are out shopping. Have a look in local markets and some craft stores. If you see something unique that you like go ahead and buy it. Your inner girl will be so happy.

Loose (or messy) Hair

Loose or messy hair occurs when the strands are not confined or pinned too much so it can hang in a freer lusty style. Bridget Bardot was famous for a sexy half-up look typical of the late 1950/60s. This involves gathering the hair at the back into an up do but leaving the sides and fringe areas to be looser. Another approach is to pull back the hair between the temples leaving the sides freer. This allows some hair to still frame your face while keeping the bulk of the weight and volume up on the head.

Loose or messy is quite a popular casual look but it also comes with a lot of subliminal messages. Loose hair is all about softness and vulnerabilities (or maybe receptiveness or open-mindedness might be better). It sends the message that you are alive to new possibilities. Messy hair on the other hand is about determination and strength. It indicates that you have a certain amount of resolve and often put others first. The emotional conflict and balance between these two is very feminine. Generally, neat pinned up hair shows poise and control and as it gets loose and comes down it implies some level of emotional overwhelm. With messy the hair starts down and goes up the more determined and focused someone is. It is not neat though because there is still that undercurrent of emotional tug-of-war driving the situation. Frayed at the edges if you will.

There are many Hollywood tropes that follow these themes from the role of women in frontier stories and spaghetti westerns, fish out of water tales, chalk-and-cheese relationships, romantic and erotic encounters through to the kick-ass, independent, action lead. Check out Madeleine Stowe in *Last of the Mohicans* and Claudia Cardinale in the controversial western *Once up a time in the West*. And for a highly charged example, Kelly McGinnis in *Witness* where eyes and hair work together. Contrast that to a more modern-day heroine in a thriller or action movie like Sigourney Weaver as Ellen Ripley in the *Alien* movies. The Jurassic Park franchise also has some good examples. Basically, these dinosaur flicks all have the same story line but work different angles from Laura Dern's idealist grad-student (Ellie Sattler), Julianne Moore's (Dr Sarah Harding) intelligent and feisty and common sense mother instinct, to Bryce Dallas Howard's (Claire Dearing) distant workaholic with a determined persona who saves the day and whose iceberg melts for a strong and difficult man. Pay attention to how the hair develops as the plot unfolds in all these movies.

When loose meets messy we often get an erotically charged or sensual appeal. This is the essence of next day hair. It is difficult to carry off for an occasional girl because the first hurdle is to be passable and then to transmit genuine feminine feelings. Loose and messy can just be an indicator that you aren't very good at dressing or that you don't really care. Or, maybe, it is just a bad hair day. Another problem is that loose meets messy also hints at bedroom hair. In more colourful language what we are talking about is that feisty but fuckable look.

You know, how you appear after 'Gladiator sex' - the passionate, rip your clothes off kind, when you are fresh from the fight, are glad to be alive, and feel strongly connected to someone. That is, like a lightning strike that grounds all that swirling emotional stuff. If you are still struggling with this, and want some kitschy fun, watch Jane Fonda in the movie *Barbarella* and you'll soon get the idea behind loose and messy.

How do you re-create this lusty lived-in look? The trick is not to do messy or loose as a go-to style but occasionally break up your normal hair look to show there is a real person inside. Follow your moods. Normally bed hair implies more mess at the back (for obvious reasons), a flaky half updo, loose ponytails or messy braids (from a bit of a tussle). So first up is not to wash your hair daily. Pile it up on top of your head to make a 'pineapple' Up Do when you are relaxing to loosen any curls and kink any straight bits. When you make a neat ponytail or a bun, go back and just tease out the hair a little from the tie or clip. Likewise, leave a stray bang or two. Pull out the odd strand from an Up Do. If your hair is straighter bring some strands together for a slightly matted effect. You can do this by letting your hair dry naturally and not comb it out too much. Muss it up by blasting the cuticles from under the hair with a dryer on light heat or massaging the base of the hair with your fingers. Then add some grittiness with a texture spray to create volume and grip.

And Finally

That is just about it for this section. In the next chapter we will look at how all the above can be used to help frame your face to make it more female. But before that, as usual, here are a few extras.

When you get your new hair, it is going to be irresistible not to try it on. You might even be tempted to wear it while you do your makeup. Don't. The big reveal when you put on your hair to complete your look is something to be savoured. Longer hair also has a habit of ending up on your face, in your mouth, or sticking to product which will ruin the moment. If you really must wear it pin it up and away from the makeup zone. A much better idea though is to start your whole routine by tidying away your own hair and putting on a wig cap/liner to leave your face and surrounding area free to work on.

General wear and tear is also something to be aware of. If you wear a human wig daily (for several hours or at work) it will last about a year. A synthetic wig has a life of about half that or four to six months. A heat friendly synthetic may last less than that if it is constantly exposed to heat treatments. Wearing a wig less will obviously increase its longevity so multiple wigs is a good idea if you can afford it. That will also give you more style options. But take care not to switch colours or style too often. Many people often regard nice girls as ones whose 'collars and cuffs' match so to speak. Constantly changing can come across a bit skanky and cheap. You don't want to be the point of discussion in the locker room or sports bar. Unless of course that is what you are after with your girl time.

We also mentioned that showering in a wig is not a good idea because it causes tangling and knotting and if you like hot showers can damage the hair fibres. The same applies if you are out and about and get caught in the rain. Either get into the dry as quick as you can or take off your wig. A sudden downpour will show up your wefts if you have that type of wig. The hair strands may also frizz when you come into the warm from the cold to dry out. Of course, if you live in a climate that is hot and humid wig maintenance is going to be an issue. There are lots of wig specific products that can help.

And last, don't be afraid to experiment. If you only keep your hair down and flat, then it is going to get very boring and samey. You might think that this is the only option for occasional dressing or to be passable. Feminization is about much more than that. When you are pottering about in your own home, cleaning, cooking, doing jobs, working from home, or choosing a change of outfit – bunch up your hair, pin it, use a loose style to keep it out of the way and feel more girly. If you have a 'girl' friend have a sleepover and braid each other's hair. Slip on some underwear, a man's shirt, and ankle socks, pile up your hair, and curl up on the sofa for a night in, watch a movie or do your nails.

Chapter 9 Framing the Face

If you already have some femme features, you may be able to get by with a nice femme hair style and the minimum of makeup. The right style can help soften and round out your face. The wrong style can make you more angular. If you dress properly and wear your hair in a female style most people will pass you as a female when they see you from the back or side profile. The careful use of curls and bangs and the shape of hair at the sides of your face all help to point to key features like your eyes and mouth. Hair can also cover features you want to hide or soften. The clever use of this negative space can give more depth and roundness to your face.

The way you wear your hair also says a great deal about your femme personality. The swish and movement of the strands, how it falls around your neck and shoulders or across your face and how you brush it away from your face, tidy it behind your ear, or control it with accessories like clips and bands will all add to your female persona. These are the themes for this chapter. What we are really talking about is how styling helps with that feminine illusion and how we use girl styles to express female emotions and psychological traits.

Best hair for your face type

Hopefully by now you have started to pick out one or two styles. It is important though that your hair style works with the shape of your face. Remember all those types we looked at in chapter 5. Let's take another look and match them up with hair.

First up are the more female shaped faces, *round, oval, and heart.* If you worked on your face shape with the makeup tips in Part 2, you probably have one of these ready to go.

Round: this face type is like a circle. The widest part of the face is by the cheekbones or the mid-ear level. The idea is to use hair styles that will complement the curve of the face by adding volume to make the overall head shape more oval. That means volume at the top and temples and/or between the chin and jaw. For short to medium you want hair styles that sweep back a little. Cuts that have layering and fullness in the crown will also be a good choice. And longer hair styles which come in under the chin and fit close to the face will make the face appear less round and longer. A bob or lob with some layering is good. Just avoid wideness only at the ears which will make you more angular or add to the roundness.

Best Options: long and layered cuts, choppy or shag pixie cut, bobs and lobs, short bangs above ears and at the sides.

Oval: if you are this shape you already have the ideal proportions. Most girl styles will work but you can gain more by focusing on a feature to frame such as your eyes, cheeks, or lips. Choose a style that brings out one of these with the side shape of the hair curving in. So forehead bangs to the eyes or an over eye side sweep, a curve in of hair between ear and jaw for the cheeks, and a turn in under or level with the chin for the mouth.

Best Options: long waves and curls, bob and lob with structure, layers, and shape

Heart: this shape has a wider more obvious forehead tapering past the cheeks to a smaller chin. We want to avoid too much volume at the top but bring the hair out between the ear and the cheek or go longer to draw out the face a little. Use a side parting and swept bangs to break up the wider forehead space. Bring in medium hair to just cover the edge of the bottom of the face and again angle longer hair to help frame the jaw line and soften the point on the chin. A layered look will also give you more shape towards the bottom of the head.

Best Options: long styles with a side-swept fringe or cut, waves and curls that start below the ear, pixie cut with a parting (if your face is already petite), bob or lob curving around the chin/jaw.

Suppose though that your face is more angular. Or, you do not want to spend time with makeup and contouring to make it softer. Then we can work with more man shaped faces as follows.

<u>Square:</u> in this shape there is no dimension to the sides with the jaw and hairline on the same vertical. Style your hair so that it has more height on top like a pouf or bouffant or even a half up do. This will make the face look longer. Short or medium hair with a bit of volume out to the sides by the ears (curls or waves) will make the face look rounder. Use ragged or curly bangs with a side parting to break up the squareness of the hair line or a mid-parting with long bangs either side like a stage curtain. Use waves or wisps of longer hair to lengthen the face but also break up or mask the stronger jaw. Avoid those Bettie Page type of straight bangs and super straight hair.

Best Options: side partings and side-swept bangs, long layered hair with some blowout or wispiness, structured bobs with layers and angle to shape and round out the middle of the head.

<u>Oblong (or rectangle):</u> this shape has length rather than width. So, we want to make it look rounder by adding some volume around the ears. A short bob will work well but angle it towards the back of the head or use a wedge cut to give you a natural line for the length of the face that fades into the jaw. For medium and chin length hair have the hair turn in under the jaw to shape or have the edges flick out which will make the face squarer (or rounder) looking. Chopped bangs down to the eyes will shorten the face while freer bangs and side partings with a bit of a sweep will break up the straight vertical. Try curvier and wavy styles with length and layering to break up that vertical between hairline and chin.

Best Options: curtain style and chopped bangs, layered cuts for volume, medium long waves or curls, wedge or angled bob, buns, or loose chignons.

The next two face types are outliers for both male and female faces. The acute angles make it tricky to balance the face but there are still lots of styling options.

Diamond: here the cheeks are very prominent, the chin can look pinched and the forehead narrow. If you have been following along with the previous choices, you will see what we need: width and height at the forehead and also some volume cheeks-to-chin. A nice full fringe with plenty of bangs will help spread out the forehead area. And layering that keeps the hair close to the head by the cheeks and then expands and curls into the chin will level up the jaw area. A bob or lob will work well as will a shag with some layering under the ears. If you go for a longer style wear it in a way that pulls back behind the ears and hangs free by the neck to give a more oblong shape. You can also do a pouf or a comb back with side bangs in a half-up look leaving some hair to dangle down the sides and hide the angle to the top of the head. Have a look at the singer/actress, *Cher*, who manages prominent cheekbones well with longer styles.

Best Options: mid to long cuts with ruffled waves, bobs and lobs from ear to chin, side partings, and ponytails (to show cheeks) with side bangs (to integrate cheeks), or chignons for a more Spanish or Latin look.

Triangles (and pear)*:* triangles are like half diamonds. So, the hair you need depends on which way the triangle points. If you have a narrow forehead than it is width and volume up top with some bangs or partings and side sweeping to make the forehead look bigger and balance up the wider jaw area. Again, hair over the ears curling or hanging back under will help soften the wider jaw. Use a bob with bangs or a more angular cut like a wedge to make the jaw a feature. A pear is similar but rounder on the cheeks so again width on the upper sides of the face to balance and wear longer hair neat at the nape to avoid the hamster look. A triangle with the width on the forehead and the point at the chin requires volume and width below the ears with hair gathered over the forehead to make it look smaller. You can do both of these things with your hair loose behind your ears and some wispy bangs, curtain style, or a side sweep over one ear. Remember the hair needs to hang either side of the jaw to compensate for the narrowness.

Best Options: layers that finish above the ear or below the ear depending on the direction of the triangle. Curl into the collarbone to frame the inverted triangle. Shag and choppy pixie cut and or short side bangs for ordinary triangle

The general principles can be summarised quite easily. Where the face is narrow compared to the cheeks add volume and width to your hair to even up the overall look of your head. Use curls and waves to break up long verticals. And layering to bring out or add shape around your existing face. Sometimes this will cover a problem and sometimes make it a feature. If you can't hide it, flaunt it. Make it look like it is there by design. Bangs can be used in a variety of ways to hide the forehead and make your face shorter or narrower or wider depending on how you part and style them. Angled and shaped bobs and lobs can absorb a sharper jaw angle by continuing the line around the back of the head.

Another trick is to use is asymmetry. It is more difficult to tell if you face is long or short or angular if you obscure it with the hair style or don't allow people to check both sides of your face. This is why longer hair pushed over one ear and left to hang over the face on the other side is such a good look. Don't hide behind your hair too much though otherwise you will come over as shy, insecure, or emo.

If you are a 24/7 girl holding down a job you cannot always go for your preferred style. You need a backup or second (quick) style that you can switch to. That is why knowing how to pin or grip your hair is such a good option. Remembering of course where you want the volume and width to end up. Arrange it like this for formal meetings and then switch to your preferred style when working in the office. Loose styles that switch between the two can work really well here and give you some feminine mystique. But too loose or messy and you will look harassed, that the job is all too much for you, or you don't care about your appearance.

Okay, so now you have an idea of what to look for in your hair pieces. It is a good idea to go back to the previous chapter and pick out a few styles that will work for you. If you haven't already, take that virtual makeover to see what they look like with and without makeup. Which ones give you the best look? Do you have enough hair to think about styling it a little with some of the techniques like pinning, bunching, braiding, or twisting to give you a few variations?

Hair and Personality

The next task is to match your chosen hair shortlist to your femme personality. Women spend an awful lot of time choosing and styling their hair in ways that match how they feel inside. If your hair is not working for you it can knock your girl confidence. And when you get that perfect look you will feel like a million dollars. Here are some typical style combinations and what psychologists and face readers reckon they say about you. Take it with a pinch-of-salt if you like but it will give you an idea of how other people might see your femme persona.

Okay, first is hair length. As we have seen very long hair is difficult to manage and is more hippie, bohemian, or typical of younger girls. The basic message is immaturity. So long hair is about freedom and/or lack of responsibility. A shorter hair style gives an indication of independence, rebelliousness, or an edgy feel. In other words, an impression that you are older, wiser, and more mature. Medium hair is in between and is a safe option that is seen as more reliable or professional. It also gives you the benefits of styling without too much time or effort.

The colour of your hair is also a marker for personal traits:

Black hair: implies you are feminine and demure. You will hold your tongue and only speak when you know your mind. As a result, you are thought of as someone that can be trusted. You are the model of propriety and elegance whether you are with strangers or friends. You project an aura of being happy and confident as well as intelligent which makes you super attractive. Silky smooth (usually long) hair is that *hime* look and is high maintenance if your hair is not naturally straight while shorter bob hair looks efficient and is easily controlled.

Blonde hair: implies you are approachable and easy going. People find it easy to talk to you. You are a down to earth kind of person and can welcome people with an easy smile. Blondes are also known for their sexy nature. A common stereotype is that blonde means less intelligent or ditsy. This, of course, is not generally true but is a feature of 'barbie' girls. Reese Witherspoon debunks this one quite effectively in the movie *Legally Blonde*. Charlize Theron gives it a sensual and savage treatment with great messy hair in *Atomic Blonde*. And, Marilyn Monroe was of course the quintessential sexy blonde bombshell. Compared to other hair colours you will find that you are approached more by males (up to 20%). This places Blondes on the needy end of the spectrum because they are used to lots of attention and are disappointed when they don't get it.

Red hair: is a sign of a burning, passionate, and fun nature. You are full of excitement and always have some goal or objective in mind but like to keep things light and good humoured. Once focused you put your heart and soul into an activity. You have good intuition and an ability to express yourself well. Such a combination marks you out for leadership roles. But be careful because you can sometimes come across as temperamental and overly feisty. You will love quickly and feverishly but can also be fickle because you enjoy the infatuation part of love but hate to be bored.

Brunette hair: signifies that you are intelligent and self-sufficient. You will find that people consult you for advice because work colleagues see you as someone who makes good decisions. You are independent though and like to do things on your own. You are street savvy and like making a difference. Brunettes are generally considered to be lower maintenance by the opposite sex compared to the other hair colours. Just as well because they account for about 60% of the population.

Irrespective of colour, people with longer hair are regarded as higher maintenance than people with shorter hair. Longer tends to imply that you are more self-absorbed and maybe a little drama queen. This is because you are more likely to spend a lot of time getting the detail right and will choose a style (or something) to get you noticed. Typically, shorter bob and pixie styles require less time on styling and use less product. This indicates that the wearers don't tend to get over fussy but also that they are less in touch with their feelings. Various studies show that women with shorter hair tend to be more intelligent, independent, and happier. Red heads with shorter hair are considered happier than red heads with longer hair. And, women with longer blonde hair are considered more attractive than blondes with shorter hair but both are considered high maintenance.

Next is the quality (texture or feel) of the hair:

Curly hair: indicates a warm-heartedness and fun-loving bubbly nature. Although there is fire, enthusiasm, and passion in this person they also have insight and intuition. This mix makes them very expressive, but they also have a difficult time focusing on long term projects. As a result, they can sometimes come across as a bit scatty or drama queen.

Wavy hair: especially when thick and glossy is a sign that a person is innovative and creative. They have high energy and a strong will to drive that innovation and get things done but they also need to feel a deep connection with projects or people. As a result, they can be hurt more than other people and will often bottle up their emotions. This means that although they can be outgoing, they also need regular time alone to recharge (especially if their hair is thinner). All that creativity also means they love to be free which can be a problem when committing to steady relationships.

Thick hair: generally, indicates strong will power, but also that you can be stubborn and immovable on issues. The thicker the hair the more energy you have to drive that will. The thinner your hair the lower will be your energy levels. In the latter you might find that you like more delicate pastimes and eschew the gym or heavier sports. Thinner hair though does tend to indicate more patience.

Straight hair: people with straight hair are considered to have a more refined personality. They are sociable, elegant, and calm but the obsession with neatness can also indicate a perfectionist who likes to be in control. These people also tend to be more outdoorsy and possibly have a low sex drive or low enthusiasm for intimate contact. If you are this type it can mean that people often will try and avoid you, that you stay late at the office, work weekends or find other ways to fill the friendship gap.

Given the above then, if you have straight hair and always try to curl or style it with more wave it can indicate that you are wanting more fun in your life. That is, if you make your hair more interesting you will tell the world that you are more fun to be with. Vice versa if you have curly or wavy hair and always try to straighten it or make it looser then it means your life is too hectic and muddled and you need to take five. By managing your hair you get a sense of control and balance.

Wash-and-go hair refers to hair that dries naturally and has the minimum of styling. If this is you then the length of your hair tells us a lot about your emotional state. Medium length indicates that you are logical, a good thinker, and competitive but you will get impatient (that is why you wash-and-go). Common sense will be important to you. You may think that people who express emotions or are a bit gushy should get over themselves. If your hair is longer you will be more romantic, chilled, creative and/or more in touch with your feelings. If you also tend to throw your hair up into loose or messy styles, or just shove it behind your ear, it indicates that you tend to put other people's needs before your own. All this implies ultra-low maintenance because it appears that you aren't focused on your own looks. It is also an indicator that not much will bother or upset you. But can be, how shall we say, mumsy, in a nice way.

The next characteristic to look at is your hairline. Female hairlines are straighter than most male ones which have an M-shape. If you only got your M shape as your hair receded, think back to how your hairline used to be because it can indicate latent feminine traits. Here are the main variations to consider:

Straight hairline: in this one the hair is horizontal across the forehead. It doesn't follow the contours of the head so it is an indicator that you might be a bit of rebel and/or a rule breaker. On a more positive note it also means that making some positive contribution to society or the world is something that you look towards.

Curved hairlines: are like little crescents which are sweet and even. This indicates that you are a 'goody two shoes' and are unlikely to misbehave or embarrass yourself. You will tend to be polite and demure at least on the outside. As they say, still waters run deep. It is likely that you did exactly what your parents or authoritative figure told you to do growing up and will expect others to also follow the rules.

Widow's peak hairlines: this shape has a downward V shape in the centre and helps form the classic heart shaped forehead. This is also the go to look for wiccans and witches. So, it says there is something enigmatic or unknown about you and hints at strange power or latent sex appeal. Like a widow you have had a taste of the bedroom and may have a secret longing for more.

Irregular hairline: is the kind that varies or undulates across the forehead. Think of it as what happens when you wrinkle your brow a lot. So, this feature is indicative of a troubled childhood or some internal struggles or conflict. It can also indicate that you did not learn about boundaries or limits growing up.

Hairlines are part of our genetics but the way we part the hair is more elective and a direct expression about our unconscious feelings:

Left side parting: indicates that you are compassionate, patient, and willing to listen to others. It means you can empathise with other people. When they are sad you can be sad with them but when you give feedback, it will be honest. A left parting will lean to a more logical, organised, and confident persona.

A right parting: indicates that you are more fun loving and emotional. You will have a more touchy-feely element and be quick with a comforting word and help when someone feels vulnerable. In a word inclusive. But you might have problems with your boundaries. You are likely to be creative but also a bit eccentric and out there.

Centre parting: or curtain style means you are a mix of the left and right styles. This means that you will be calm and reliable but also have a fun side too. You can mix the logical with the emotional and keep things in proper balance. So, in a word, charming. However, you can also come across as a social butterfly and a bit short on solid convictions.

No Parting: indicates a good mixture of left and right brain activities but someone who is also low maintenance. It is that fuss-free thing again. This though can be interpreted as a casual attitude so you might find that people ignore you when it comes to social events (think wall flower) or walk all-over you in meetings or otherwise to get what they want.

Random parting: If you find that your hair just happens to fall into some kind of random parting especially when your hair is loose, depending on your mood, or when you wash-and-go this can indicate you get bored easily, are opinionated, or just like to be animated. Other people may see you as a bit unpredictable or unreliable.

The approach you take to cutting your hair (rather than style it) can also reveal things about you. For example:

Blunt cuts: are more angular and like shorter hair indicate a no nonsense attitude. This is a low maintenance style and it probably means you are focused and want to get things done. You won't suffer fools gladly and expect people to jump to your tune.

Layered cuts: are very neat. They control the hair and make it look just so. They may reflect your ordered life. You probably have a place for everything in your closet and like everything in its place. In fact, you are a bit of perfectionist. You have that eye for detail and will not like it your hair gets frayed or out of place.

Waved cuts: neat hair with a hint of a wave or more vintage style have a hint of mystery or scandal. You will tend to be captivating and or appealing to people and will draw them towards you. Think of those finger wave hair dos in Agatha Christie mysteries. In short, a bit of charisma or animal magnetism. Looser Surfer Girl waves are all about confidence and energy. Apart from the bravery associated with paddling out to meet the big wave you like to be with family and friends, but welcome strangers too. Think night barbeques on the beach. You will speak with conviction and be admired for it. You like your freedom and independence and a little alone time sometimes too.

Unconventional cuts: mix all types of colouring and styles including undercuts and shaves. They say you are creative and fun to be with. Probably you are an artist or have artistic tendencies and think outside the rules. You also like to be carefree and ride the emotional rollercoaster. This can make you capricious and difficult to be with. You will probably be the first on anyone's invite list –to see what you will get up to or just to liven things up. Think Lady Gaga, Madonna, and Rihanna.

Now you might think, since you are not really a girl, how can all this possibly apply to you. Well here are three ways that all this can help. First, is to link up with your inner girl. Quite often you will find that she is psychologically quite different to your male persona. So have a conversation with her and decide what kind of traits she has then go through the lists and match up the various characteristics to build a hair style for her. Second if you are being feminized by a partner you might appreciate more of what she is wanting when she dresses you. You can take that more passive role by adopting some of the behaviours associated with your girl type. Another thing you can do is to pay attention to your partner's hair and see what it says about her personality. You might appreciate why more dominant women tend to have carefully coiffured hair, like perfect layers, straight long hair, bobs or lobs, short blunt cuts, straight bangs, or ponytails. If her hair is softer, she may lean more towards a velvet domme personality and more domestic styles of play. Knowing these things will help bring you closer together in your relationship.

When you finally connect your hair to your inner girl there will be a fantastic moment. You will know she is you and you are her. So do take some time and effort to pick the right style and cut. Repeat that mindfulness exercise at the start of the book and check out how your Anima hair appears. This fusion will be especially important if you are a 24/7 girl or in transition. Even if you remain sceptical about all this remember that all the above will be used unconsciously by other people when they interact with you. If you do not connect with the girl inside the persona will not be congruent with the outside presentation and that can be a very big tell even if your makeup is perfect.

Age Appropriate Hair

Okay, time for something different. Hair has a fascinating history and has long been used to differentiate gender by length and style. Ideas about the appropriate hair length for males and females have been heavily influenced by religion and culture. In certain eras women's hair has been covered or bound in various ways especially after marriage. This custom is still observed in weddings when bridal hair comes with a veil or elaborate decoration. Sometimes these persuasions have also found their way into law. In colonial times in the United States some areas passed laws saying that a woman's hair belonged to her husband and she wasn't allowed to cut it unless the husband gave permission. In the Roman Empire, ladies of the night were required to have blonde or fair hair. They dyed it with all sorts of ash and powders which is where the idea of the ash or platinum blonde come from.

In the Regency period wearing the hair up and decorating it with ornaments and ribbons often in romantic designs was popular until looser styles like poufs and curls reappeared in Victorians times. We have the latter to thank for our current ideas about correctness and hair length. Overly loose adult hair was seen as having sexual connotations while freer longer styles with pigtails and ponytails were considered juvenile. The Edwardian cute girl look is now heavily copied in Lolita fashion made popular in Japanese subculture. Pinned up adult hair though has become a mark of propriety and correctness.

The convention in Victorian times was that girls would stop wearing their hair down and put it up in braids when they moved into their late teens and early womanhood or came out as debutantes. After that the hair would be worn in more elaborate Up Dos especially after marriage to show sobriety, correctness, and respectability. This culminated in the Gibson Girl look which we most associate with Victorian ladies in period dramas. Hence the phrase 'letting your hair' down when you are being freer or a little naughty or raunchy. The idea that hair should be more circumspect, controlled, short (or up) as you mature continues to this day.

The pre-Raphaelite movement seriously challenged these Victoria ideals and became very controversial and risqué. The reference subjects for art works were often modelled on the wives and mistresses of bohemian artists and appeared in paintings of partially clad figures in depictions of Roman and Greek fables. The look consisted of pale skin, willowy bodies, scarlet lips, exceptionally long flowing hair, and sulky or melancholic expressions. The pre-Raphaelites considered this more realistic than the more circumspect pictures of the artist Raphael which were approved by the establishment of the time. Wearing flowers and garlands in the hair was also linked to paganism. The first woman, Eve, is often depicted in this style with long flowing hair and just a few fig leaves for cover. Eve, of course, reputably lured Adam into sinful ways. And womankind has been sort of paying for it ever since.

Tips for Mature hair

A woman is regarded as mature when she reaches the age of 32 (42 for men). Maturity generally means a whole bunch of personality traits which show that you are more balanced and accepting of the world around you. For example, you are able to keep long term commitments, are not as affected by flattery or criticism, can make decisions based on character not emotion, consistently recognise other people's contribution to your life and success with appropriate expressions of gratitude, think before acting, and can prioritise the needs of others over yourself.

Because your life is more balanced this means that hairstyles and makeup also settle into something more consistent that defines your character rather than being led by fads and fashions. That is good news because it means that you will not need to buy as many hair pieces or mix up your look too often. And, practice will make perfect. To reflect this different stage of your life there are some key characteristics to try and capture in your appearance: a natural look, professional but also fashionable, low-maintenance, bold and shaggy, edgy with a touch of sportiness, sophisticated and sexy, elegant and stylish.

A shorter hair cut will help to flatter your face by focusing on the stronger facial features such as the cheekbones where the skin does not sag as you age. The trick is to make a layer of hair that shows your jawline if it is still well defined but softer than when you were younger or to bring the hair out at the cheeks. Long bobs, shaggy styles, and wavy hair are the way to go. As you move into your 50s you can take a shorter pin straight style. Bangs also become more important because they will cover up any wrinkles on your forehead and compensate for any receding hairline. This will knock years off your face. Hair also gets thinner as we age so this needs to be reflected with layers to lighten thicker hair and to create finer hair.

As you get older movement becomes more restricted so you need something that is simple and easy unless you can afford a stylist. A tint or rinse can help style the Gray but don't overdo it with shocking shades. Longer hair as we have seen is mostly out unless it is kept up, but you can get away with medium lengths with a bit of care. Long hair tends to lengthen the face especially when it is offset with looser skin around the jowl area. Very straight long hair will make this look worse. And the weight of hair will be more difficult to carry and manage. All this is does not sound very appealing but can be offset with shaping and layering of the hair at the sides.

Here are eight useful ways to help your mature hair (pieces) look more authentic:

Short hair: is better with lots of dimension so what you want is hair with highlights. These tick several of the boxes above. For example, pixie cuts or a feathered or shaggy bob. See row one of Figure 14 (last chapter).

Hint at aging gracefully: by adding lowlights. These are the opposite of highlights and make your hair appear darker. For example, if you are blonde add some darker caramel or honey colour to give you a dirty blonde look. Likewise tint a grayer wig a little darker brown or black to hint at your original hair colour. Needs to be done with care though so use a stylist. This will give you the sexy appeal of a Mrs Robinson (aka the movie, *The Graduate*).

Use a warmer hair colour (like brown or golden blonde): try some caramel to make your complexion glow more and add youth. With a shaggy or sassy or even a curly French style bob cut this will also look sporty. A short boho (or bohemian) style might work if your hair is thicker or you still want it longer.

For wavy or curly hair: balayage– this means hand painting highlights onto the curls to give a more natural sun-kissed or bleached look. It is different to normal highlights because the colour is less uniform. This will look as though your hair is naturally losing its colour. Try this with a short or medium style with curly bangs swept off the face.

Choose hair with more volume so that it does not hang limp or fall over your head. If you are using your own hair add more volume with hair product and/or a little blow out. Youthful hair has more body particularly at the crown.

Look for hair with a bit of a sheen. Shiny glossy hair is an indicator of youthful well-nourished hair but not too much or it will look false. This is doubly true if you are purchasing a synthetic hairpiece for your look. Cheap lower quality ones have more shine.

Hint that you dye: *the* older you get the more hair tends to be grayer or white. So, if your hair piece doesn't have these colours it can look too youthful and out of place. Use the colour you want but add shadows on the roots to give a hint that you dye.

Go with gray: acknowledge your age. Keep the gray alive though with some careful tinting, highlighting, and lowlighting to give variation. Too much and it will look metallic and silver, so keep it real. If the hair is straight don't make it too sleek but do keep it neat.

If you want to see how all this works in practice checkout the following celebrities who have mastered the secret of aging gracefully: Cindy Crawford, Helen Mirren, Julianne Moore, Meryl Streep, Christy Turlington, Halle Berry, Julia Roberts, and Jane Fonda to name a few.

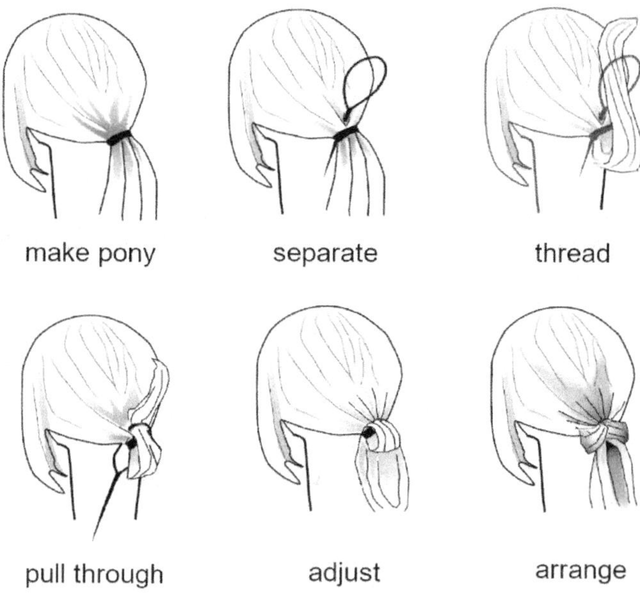

Figure 15 Using a ponytail loop

Topsy Tail Styles

Whether you are young or more mature one way to look elegant without too much effort is a topsy-tail styling. For these you will need an accessory called a hair or ponytail loop. Basically, this is a flexible oval shape with a rat tail. The idea is that you make a ponytail and then use the hair loop to form an elegant twist and tie.

There are lots of ways that you can style your hair using this method but here are a few easy ones to get you going:

The flipped pony: gather your hair in a low ponytail. Secure with an elastic hair tie. Separate the hair above the tie by using the tail of the hoop. Stick it in your hair so the tail separates the hair and the loop is sticking up vertically (see Figure 15). This frees your hands. Take hold of the ponytail and thread it through the hoop. Take hold of the hoop tail and pull the hoop and ponytail through the gap in the hair. Arrange it as tight or as loose as you want to give a gentle twist at the top of the ponytail. In the last step either you can gather second bunches either side of the main ponytail and pull through again or just tease out the sides of the ponytail to give more body.

Hidden pony: in this one you use your hair to hide the hair tie, so it looks like your ponytail is tied by your hair. Make a ponytail and tie off with a hair tie. Use a small hoop (they come in different sizes). Insert the tail of the hoop to separate the pony behind the tie (just like above). Take a gather of hair from one side of the ponytail. Wrap it around the base to cover the hair tie. Feed the end of the gather back through the hoop. Pull the hoop through the gap to tie off the hair.

Chignon pony: make a loose ponytail just above the nape. Use the hoop tail to separate out the hair behind the tie. Thread the hair through the hoop and pull through like before. Now repeat the process. Tie off the remaining part of the ponytail. Separate with the hoop tail, thread, and pull through. Now you have two pretty twists. Leave as is or wrap the excess ponytail and tuck under the twists and secure with bobby pins. Use clips or grips if you want to accessorise further.

Side Pony: leave your hair down and part to one side. Make a ponytail on the side of the head next to the parting. Separate with the hoop tail. Flip and pull through like before. Now you have a lovely twist on the side above the ear. Secure the rest of the ponytail however you like, leave it free, or repeat the above for extra twists.

Loose Pony: for this one, make the first ponytail high up on the head. Separate, flip, and pull through. Secure the twist with pins or whatever. Choose a place further down the remaining pony and tie off. Separate, flip, and pin. Repeat the process until you reach the end of the ponytail and then secure it under the last flip. Obviously, you get different looks depending on how tight or loose you make the twists and how separated the ties are on the ponytail.

Braided Pony: for this one form a ponytail as before. Separate the hair into two gathers below the hair tie and braid each one separately (like a fish tail). Insert the hoop tail above the hair tie. Thread the braids through the hoop. Pull the tail and hoop through to form a braided twist. Alternatively take one of the braids and wrap it around the tie and then pass through the loop and pull through. This will give a braided tail with a braid wrap for a hidden look.

Twin Pony: for this separate the hair at the back and make two ponytails like Odango style except lower and on the back of the head. Apply one of the above techniques to one tail and then to the other. Join them together at the bottom by wrapping the remaining tails under the final twist and securing with pins and accessorise with clips and grips.

As you can see there is a lot of scope so be as inventive as you like and have fun. A basic two-piece loop set with a large and junior hoop costs £/$2-3 and an accessory set with additional clips less than £/$5 so very affordable and lots of bang for your buck. Alternatively make your own with a piece of thin plastic. Bend it over into a loop and then tape the ends together to create the tail. Make a large and small one.

Pencil or stick hair

Another chic look that has that loose unkempt but stylish appeal is pencil or stick hair. For this one you use a pen or a pencil so you can do it in the office or anywhere where you have something to hand. The key point is that there are no grips or ties involved so the hold comes from the twist and tension in the hair itself.

Figure 16 illustrates the process. First gather your hair into a loose ponytail. It helps if you twist the hair around clockwise a few times to create some tension and then hold it in your left hand. With your right hand, position the pencil or stick horizontally a little away from your head and fold the pony over. Now wrap the ponytail clockwise around the base until all the hair is used. It looks neater if you tuck in the tail of the hair and helps with hold. Next hold the hair in place and rotate the stick, until it is between a 12 o'clock and 2 o'clock position. You might want to go fully around once or twice until you are happy with the tension. Don't make it too tight or the next step will be difficult but too loose and it won't hold. Now flip the stick over vertically and away from your head. Twist the hair as you fold it back and push the stick into the hair for better hold. Make any adjustments you feel necessary for comfort and look.

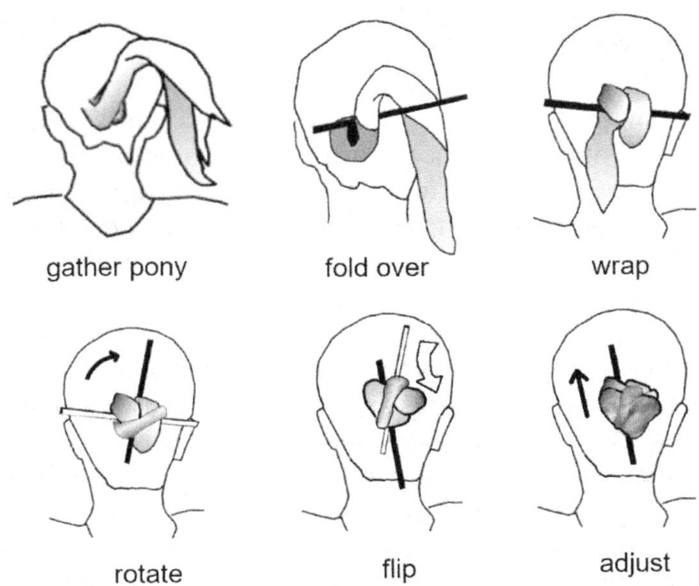

Figure 16 Pencil (or stick) hair

Once you get this down you can use anything that is pencil or stick shaped and firm like chopsticks or decorated wooden sticks or even a stick with a clasp for a more deliberate chic look. Nice wooden sticks with a leather clasp look great with mature grey hair. Plain craft sticks are also available that you can decorate yourself. If you keep the tension looser then you can also create a quick messy hair style.

Stick hair has been around for thousands of years, in many different cultures from ancient to modern. The current popularity is due to Japan where *Kanzashi* refers to a whole range of rigid hair ornaments. And, in Korea, the term *binyeo* refers to fixing chignons with decorative and ornate sticks. So, if you like this look there is a whole world to discover. Once you master the single stick approach try the double stick or 'knitting needle' style.

Putting it all together

Okay, let's spend a little time making sense of all the above. The first and most important thing is to think about your hair style and how this matches your face and personality. After that you can accessorise and match up your clothes and jewellery as much or as little as you want.

Have a conversation with your inner girl and ask her what she wants. The more authentic you are the more passable and natural your look will be. There are a few mobile and online apps out there which will allow you to play with hair styles. Now you know the names and what they mean you can click through and try different hair pieces. Take that virtual makeover. List out the different options and styles for your personality and then shortlist. If you have two or three styles that is more than enough. Once you know what you want search online for different types of hair pieces and order as many as you need or book a trip to a stylist. It is also a good idea to have a backup style which uses clips, grips, and pins to give a slight variation on your main style. This allows you a little more spontaneity so you can put your hair up when you are on-the-go which will add to your overall authenticity as well as being practical, especially if you have longer hair which is likely to dangle and get in the way.

A couple of further ideas for longer problematic side hair or bangs is to do a quick gather. For this look just take the few strands that are constant offenders in that they get in your face, stuck to your lips, or in your mouth while you are eating, and just pull them back either side of the head and clip them round the back. Keep them loose rather than tight and they will look extra pretty but will not get in your way. If you are younger think about twisting or braiding them in a loose way. Alternatively, push the hair over your ear and pin in the side while you are eating or working. It is incredible how just doing this will make you feel so much more femme.

We looked at hair accessories in the last chapter and a lot of these are functional aids to getting the right style but they can also be used as distractors by choosing the right colours or a bit of detail like a pretty bow, a pearl finish, flowers or butterflies. So even if you don't need it for a style you can still add in a clip, a slide, or a pin to lift the observers eye away from your face or an area that might be a tell. Just add them where we concentrated the hair in the above sections. If you can give your hair some flick, bounce, blowout or movement by making it wispy or light it will present a moving target which will prevent the observers eyes from being able to scan and look for tells. Especially if you are demonstrative, bubbly, lively in movement or conversation. It is that old magician's trick of distraction again. Not too much though or that will make you look skittish and nervous.

The key is to balance your overall hair arrangement. The French aristocrat, Marie Antionette, was known for many excesses but a particular one was big hair. She pioneered *Le pouf* and piled it in elaborate up dos several feet high and added lots of ornaments like little castles and boats. The fashion for powdered and highly decorated wigs followed. That was all over-the-top, literally. You don't want to emulate that and look more like a caricature than a real person. Subtle is better.

And finally

We are nearly done with hair but again there a few things you should know about body language and hair touching. Men will tend to groom their hair behind closed doors. Females are more likely to do it in public and especially when talking to others. Playing with your hair is a sign of personal grooming which means that either you want to draw attention to or need to comfort yourself. What we are talking about is twisting, tossing, flicking, combing, wrapping, examining, or running the fingers through the hair. Some women also suck, smell, or stroke their hair which is an unconscious substitute for a pacifier. We won't pursue that one. Don't suck or smell your hair okay.

Traditionally women are not allowed or encouraged to verbalise how attracted they are to someone or for that matter how available or sexually needy they are. If you do that you will get the reputation of a dirty girl or an easy lay. So instead females have a ton of suggestive non-verbals. Here are the main ones associated with hair. If you really connect with your inner girl then all these gestures will come out so learn to read the signs of what she is telling you and others.

Touching and ruching: when a woman plays with her hair it creates movement. Movement is designed to grab attention. In nature visual systems are often keyed only to movement so rearranging your hair is an ancient way to wave a flag and let someone know you are here. Adjustment is a way of primping to say look how pretty and attractive I am. Once you have their attention you can start to use other body language and eye techniques.

Hair tossing/flipping involves flicking the hair over your shoulder or off the face. It shows the volume and thickness of your hair and how shiny it is. This is a sign of health and vitality. Be careful though because an aggressive hair toss can also mean that you feel threatened and want to make yourself (or your mane) bigger to ward off predators. Sometimes the hair is pulled up and away from the neck and into a temporary bun or ponytail before being let go to fall back. This does two things it shows how luxurious your hair is and also exposes your most vulnerable parts (the neck and boobs, if the hair is longer) showing you are passive and open. In other words, approachable. It can also be a sign of tiredness or stiffness so it depends very much on the context. If eye-contact comes with it then it's an attractor.

Twisting happens when a stray strand or bunch of hair is pulled loose and twirled around a finger. This is often unconscious and can have two meanings. First it is a kind of pacifier to soothe current feelings for example in a boring situation or when someone is engrossed in a film or magazine. But it can also be used as an attractor and indicate that you are available and/or seeking attention. Ringlets are often worn by younger prim women so it is hints at innocence but curly hair also suggests a passionate and fun person. So, twisting can reveal an unconscious desire that you want to be naughty. The difference is whether or not twirling is used with eye-contact. No eye contact indicates soothing or boredom. With eye contact and/or a coy smile it is a sexual cue.

Inspecting the hair. You will also see women pulling strands of hair loose and then examining the ends. This is mainly an act of boredom and designed to distract, soothe, or calm the individual. Actually, they may be examining the ends for fray or splitting and may even run their fingers through their hair to comb or detangle. These are all self-grooming activities. If a woman does it while you are talking to them, she thinks something better will come along. This is most certainly a brush-off signal.

Hair tidying such as combing, brushing, gathering, and adjusting bangs etc are all signs of preparing to say look I'm neat and tidy and attractive. These may be done in public just before being introduced to someone or as a female group preening activity. It is rarely done in front of a male. So, when a woman touches her hair like this in male company it is an attraction signal. In conversations a female shows that she is interested, shy, or nervous and maybe having a butterfly-in-the-tummy moment by brushing bangs to the side, tucking hair behind the ear, or otherwise just touching the hair lightly. Such behaviour may also be accompanied by a smile, brief eye-contact, a demure look away, a flush or a combination of the above. Mostly they are all unconscious signals that she likes what she sees.

Open or closed hand. If a woman adjusts the hair off her face with the hand turned so the palm is hidden, it usually indicates uncertainty, shyness, or just that she is absorbed in what she is doing. The more frequent the gesture the more likely it is to be associated with nerves or anxiety. If she sweeps hair away with the palm facing outwards, it is more of a come-on signal. Because it exposes the inside wrist which is another vulnerable area. Check eye contact for confirmation.

The neck tilt. the neck is one of our most vulnerable areas, it is the place a big cat will target to land a kill – hence the phrase 'go for the jugular'. The neck can be exposed by sweeping, flipping, or wrapping the hair away from the neck. Neck exposure like this says 'look, I'm open'.

Likewise, if a woman covers her neck or tries to protect it with hair or a hand then she is feeling threatened and telling you to back off. The neck tilt is a powerful variant on this where a female plays with her hair and tilts the neck to 45 degrees to expose the flesh. She might also stroke her neck to draw attention to it. This is a submissive signal that says, 'come and get me; I won't put up a fight.' The inherent symbolism in this is what makes all those vampire flicks so erotically charged.

So, if you want to appear more authentic learn some of these moves. Practice in front of the mirror to coordinate your hair and eye moves so they look natural. When you are en-femme just notice whether you are more prone to hair touching. Do you find yourself twirling when you are relaxing, watching a movie or reading? How often do you touch or expose your neck? Does it happen when you are around particular people? And, spare a thought for our poor male colleagues. A little flirting is okay, but no one likes a tease, darling. Especially not a prick tease. If you are not looking for that kind of involvement do not lead someone on. Use your femme powers wisely.

Chapter 10 Loose Ends

Styling your jewellery and accessories to match your face and hair is another feminine skill to acquire. Doing this correctly can make or break your look and depends on your hair, your face shape, and the length and thickness of your neck. Although you can use other decorated accessories such as clips, slides, and bows in the rest of your hair as distractors or points of interest what we are talking about here are things that can work on or close to your face.

We will cover four things. First is ear jewellery showing you what is available and how to match it to your hair to help balance your look and give you an extra boost. Next, we will consider chokers and what they can say about your personality. After that are glasses and contact lenses. Although being a bit foggy-eyed can be adorably ditsy for a short time you really need to be able to wear your formula lenses to function properly. You cannot wear contacts all the time so girl-glasses are a must. We will show you the difference between boy and girl frames and choose ones that match your face type.

Last, but not least, if you are struggling with matching your hair colour to your eye colour or want to wear a certain shadow, you can choose contact lenses for the perfect colour combo. Increasing your pupil size will also help to give you a more feminine look. When you combine that with extra big and intensely coloured irises you can create a doll-eye look which is popular on the club circuit and for anime cosplay. Alternatively, they can help disguise your appearance if you are concerned about being recognised.

Ear Jewellery

Before we get into the details it is worth saying that for a more authentic feel it is better to have your ears pierced. This way you will still be able to feel girly even when you are not en-femme and will be able to wear a wider variety of fashion jewellery when you are. Until you have worn a lovely pair of earrings and felt them dangle about your face you cannot really say you are complete crossdresser. Indeed, picking out some nice jewellery to wear, holding them up to your ears, and checking out your look should be an essential part of your makeup routine.

It is now more acceptable for men to pierce their ears so you can always wear man studs or a more aggressive something when you are not en-femme. The usual piercing is in the ear lobe, but you can also pierce other parts of the ear. Multiple piercings per ear will give you more choice and an edgier look but the more feminine multiples are confined to the lobe and ear helix. If that route is a no-no because of work restrictions or because your dressing is a secret, there are other solutions that do not involve piercings. Either way, there is no need to miss out on this most feminine of activities.

Basically, you have a choice of three styles: minimal, statement, and body piercing stuff that is used as jewellery. The latter involves barbells, bead rings, flesh tunnels, and plugs. Besides glitzy jewellery you can use other things, like cuffs and chains but unless you are going for a more tribal, ethnic, or edgy look these can be a little in your face. For example, a nose ring or a cute little jewel stud have feminine qualities but do attract more attention to where you might have contoured your nose. Likewise, a nose to ear chain can be full of eastern promise. And, if that is not for you, elaborate ear chains (or the Bajoran look) can be very eye catching. Bajorans are also worn by men and so can have an androgynous feel. The Bindi look uses jewellery on your forehead and brow region. This a popular bridal look in India but more recently has been popularised by the likes of Gwen Stefani. Anyway, for simplicity and the fact that we are more into the softer femme side of things in this book we will not consider these any further.

Here is the usual A-Z so we know what we are talking about:

Minimal earrings are referred to as studs. The stud is basically a small gemstone, plastic ball, or metal design on the end of a post. The post slots through the ear piercing and is fastened at the back with a clutch that slides on. For more expensive stones the post can be threaded allowing the back to screw on. You can also get lockable earrings that have latches or levers. Sometimes the post can have a tray attachment so more stones can be added and appear to float on the ear. These are referred to as climbers or crawlers. A Huggy is a smaller plain ring that sits close to the ear and is mainly used for piercings that are not on the main earlobe. Sometimes they might have a little decorative ball attached to hide the join. Buttons, domes, and flat disks are also popular. Studs are simple but classy and often an easy choice for work or just to keep the piercing open.

Statement earrings: as the name suggests are bolder both in colour and design. There are four main types: dangles, hoops, tassels, and sparkles.

Dangles do what the name suggests they hang from the earlobe using a thin piece of wire arranged in a hook shape. The hook goes through the piercing so the earring can 'dangle' and sometimes has a little clip to keep them in place. If there is no clip and the wire bends back slightly it is referred to as a French hook. These types use tension to keep them in place and do not pull your ear so much. A fishhook design has a circle at the end of the hook that is used to attach the decorations. Various designs and materials can be added to the wire for different effects. The length can vary from just under the earlobe (referred to as drops - like a dew drop pearl) to long ones that reach the shoulders (for example an ostrich eye or feather look). Obviously, the more weight the more likely they are to stress your ear and pull the lobe. There is a definite girly appeal to them though as they swish with your movement.

Hoops are circles, semi-circles, or arc shapes. Usually they are made of thin metal tubing. For full circles, the hoop is hollow and has a join. The join is filled with a thinner piece of metal or wire. The hoop is opened, the thin piece threaded through the piercing, and then joined back together for a seamless look. Sleeper rings are tiny plain hoops that fit through the piercing and are often worn at night or just after first piercing to keep the hole open. Semi-circles normally come with a French hook style and arcs can have a post like a stud with a clutch. The hoops can be embellished and decorated in various ways and can also form the base for a dangle. The arc style may include a tray for gemstones to be inserted so they curve under the ear.

Tassels are basically any material that forms a tuft or bunch of loosely hanging threads gathered or knotted at one end. The gathered end is fastened to a hook or a post to attach to the ear. The knot can be a small ball or a real knot of material. The threads can be any form of dangle including hoops. A rod or plate can be used to carry other decorations like beads or set stones. If there is just one thread or plate it is just a dangle. The length varies and depends largely on the weight the earlobe can take. There are so many styles that you are bound to find something you like.

Sparkles: can be hoops, dangles, tassels, or stud combinations whose main job is to catch the light. They are a bit like glitterballs except for your ears. An extension to the simple drop is a chandelier which opens out into multiple drops with lots of stones. Multiple teardrops can be stacked vertically in a dangle. Fancier versions might have a cluster of stones arranged in a decorative pattern like a flower, butterfly, bow, or S-shape. A Jacket version is a stud with an extra vertical attachment on the post like a bar or a fan that allows stones to frame the ear lobe so that they appear to float under the rim of the ear.

<u>Options for non-pierced ears:</u> if you like the idea of ear jewellery but are a bit squeamish when it comes to piercing or it is not compatible with the rest of your life you can still enjoy dressing your ears. Clip-on or spring clips first appeared in the 1930s and had quite a following until pierced ears came back into fashion during the 1980s. Basically, the back of the earring holds a small grip which uses tension to hold onto the ear. A variation is a screw form that allows you to adjust the tension on the clip. A more modern innovation are magnetic earrings which give a more realistic look and are almost indistinguishable from pierced ones. Basically, the back (clutch part) and the front are made of magnetic materials that attract one another. They sandwich your earlobe so look very authentic. Spring hoops that have a cut in the circle but are tensioned so that they can grip on to either side of the ear are also available.

The problem with all of the above is that the squeezing on the ear can make them sore if you wear them for too long. Stick-ons are like stud earrings but the back of the decoration has sticky pad that attaches to the front of the lobe. They might last you for a party but otherwise not worth the effort. Large hook earrings build on the French idea and fit over your whole ear gripping the back allowing the earring to dangle by the ear lobe. A more realistic variation is a hook that hangs over the ear but ends just inside the ear next to the ear lobe with a circle that can be used to attach other earring pieces.

Health and Hygiene: before you jump in, there are a few things to know about getting your ears pierced. First, you will have to wear something constantly to keep the holes open. Piercings less than six months old will close within 24 hours which is why you need to wear sleepers and/or studs even if you are not glammed up or en-femme. Second, there is a good (33%) chance you will have complications at some point. Issues range from ear infections, to body reactions such as granulomas, keloids, and allergies.

If your femme hygiene routine is good and you keep the posts and hooks clean and wash your ears regularly you should not have too many problems. Granulomas occur when your immune system does not like the interference and tries to wall off that bit of the body. This is more likely with multiple piercings and if you pierce the ear cartilage and not just the lobe. Keloids occur when the body creates extra scar tissue which can become much bigger than the original size of any cut or piercing. Allergies are more likely if you react to the metals or materials in the posts and hooks or areas that touch your skin. Do not be put off by all this though. Millions of women have their ears done with no problems. Just avoid constantly wearing heavy earrings or yanking them about or catching them when they are in. All these things are more likely to generate a reaction. In fact, so many women have their ears pierced that it will be a kind of tell if you remain a plain Jane. So, at the very least you will need some simple/plain studs, buttons, or dome earrings even if they are clip-ons or magnetic ones.

You can buy fashion earrings cheaply at most accessory shops in small packs. At first you are better with costume jewellery which is super cheap to mid-range ($/£ 3-5 per set). The trays and so forth are coated plastic and you can get sparkle with diamante and other inexpensive stones. Remember, diamonds are a girl's best friend. But don't neglect the other gemstones too!

There are also lots of TV sales channels that auction or offer super quality and cheap jewellery that will make you look a million dollars. Again, you need to work out what you want to complement your face and hair before you dive into purchases. At least now you know what to look out for.

Jewellery and your face type

Just like hair, earrings can work with your face type. Hooped earrings will always make your face look rounder so if you are not a standard girl shape (round, oval, or heart) they can be a good choice. Long dangling earrings give the face more length so good for girl shaped faces but not so good for longer oblong faces. The right size and shape of earring can also help balance a diamond, triangle, or even heart shape face by filling the void under the ear next to the cheek. But if your earrings are too big or have too much dazzle, they will diminish your face making all your features look smaller. Below are some suggestions for different face types but do mix and match to create a look all of your own:

Round: use angular earrings such as triangles to break up the roundness. Longer earrings like dangles will make your face appear longer (or more oval). A chandelier will frame the jaw quite nicely and sparkles will make the face glow.

Oval: use any style you want but avoid too much length. Sparkle studs will light up your face and button studs are demure but still classy.

Heart: drop earrings and short dangles will help frame the smaller chin. Use jackets to frame the ear and widen the lower face.

Square: hoops are the thing. Counteract the right-angle shape of the jaw with arcs. Huggies, creepers, and jackets will look nice too. Think about disks or crescent moons and other styles with curves. You might think a dangle will help hide the jaw, but it will just make the face look wider.

Oblong and Rectangle: avoid anything that dangles or is too vertical. A larger hoop will also emphasis face length. Use earrings close to the ear such as gemstone studs, jackets, and arcs under the ear lobe. Larger buttons will widen the face and pull up the chin. Smaller moon crescents and disks will also work.

Diamond and Triangles: dangles with long plates, thin verticals, or tassels to offset the cheekbones and fill the void as the face angles in towards the jaw. A chandelier can also look gorgeous especially if you leave the hair off your face. For a wider jaw triangle use studs and minimal choices.

The trick with these variations is to consider the size and colour of the earrings. A metallic sparkle can have just as much effect with a small earring as a plainer larger choice. Demonstrative colours and patterns can really complement your face and make a statement about personality. Too large however and they will distract from your face (which is maybe what you want). Too small and the face and hair will need to support your look. Earrings like dangles and tassels have their own momentum so can act as an attracter or distracter when you move around a room. Learn how to work your look by drawing attention or distracting to control another's focus. For example, brushing away or tidying your hair over your ear to show off your earrings when you lean forward, bend or are in conversation.

Jewellery that works with your hair

Another aspect to consider is jewellery that matches the length and style of your hair.

Short hair: in this case your hair is going to have less body, possible angles, asymmetric undercut or shave, so it is likely that the hair will be off your ears or expose more of the ear than just the lobe. Studs and other earrings close to the ear will look fantastic. Jackets, arcs, creepers and crawlers will all be good especially with small pearls, runs of pearls or for more formal occasions gemstones. You can also use huggy rings for multiple piercings on the helix of the ear. Anything that dangles or is too hooped will distract from your face and that clean shaped look.

Medium (to shoulder length) hair: in this case the bottom of the hair creates a line that marks the end of your head and face -especially if it is a straight horizontal cut. Because the hair rests or catches on the shoulders it will tend to bow outwards as you move your head up and down or from side to side. These natural movements can leave a gap that exposes your earlobes. So, what you need is something with a bit of dangle but also a bit of body and sparkle to fill the void – aka drops, tassels, and chandeliers. The trick though is to avoid earrings that are close to or lower than your shoulders or too wide otherwise they will get tangled and/or elongate your face.

Curly hair: is more wayward and its movement can catch in your earrings and get tangled. The best option is therefore earrings that stay close to your ear. That is studs, clusters, buttons, jackets, and arcs. Sparkles can complement the curls but plainer ones that work with and complement your hair colours are good too. A hoop is not out of the question but use bigger, plain, metallic ones which are easier to detangle.

Hair down: when your hair hangs down past your ears it will compete with your earrings so the simplest thing to do is go elegant and simple with minimal earrings or studs. Give them a little jazzle by choosing a gemstone that you like or that matches your eye colour or the rest of your makeup. For a classier look go with simple pearl studs either as singles or as little clusters. Clusters with a pearl or gemstone in the centre or a Jacket style to frame the lobe are very sweet. Of course, you can also use fancier (or statement) pieces but think about how they balance your face.

Chignons and low Buns: here the hair is gathered at the nape or slightly to one side. This exposes your neck and shoulders. Choose understated earrings that fit close to the ear but with a little dangle and/or sparkle. A drop pearl or gemstone is ideal. And if you want to glam it up use a precious coloured stone circled by diamonds. The dangle will also work with any loose or softer (or baby) hair at the base of your neck.

Up dos and high Buns: here the hair is pulled way off your shoulders and will expose a lot of your ear. So, you need to use the earrings to compensate for the lack of hair. You can do this spectacularly though because the earring will be visible from more angles than with your hair down. What you want are long thin dangles, showy tassels and hoops. Use plainer pattern designs for everyday and then really wow when you are out socialising with some sparkles. For formal events wheel out the statement pieces with precious metals and gemstones and diamonds.

Half up and Half down: shows off longer hair bangs so you need to work with the side framing. The trick is not to overstate your earrings – so studs again. Sparkles will look classy but more plain colours can give you an everyday chic look. Just don't make them too big or long.

Ponytails and bunches: need different earrings depending on the height of the ponytail. If the pony is fixed or cuffed high on the head, you can show of your ears and balance the sides of your face in the same way as an Up Do. If your ponytail is mid head or more braid like and demure the earrings should be understated – so studs, buttons, and maybe some classy gemstones. If you are more casual with side pigtails or doggy ears which are more juvenile stick with simple plain earrings and studs, not expensive jewellery. Dangles and hoops can get tangled with longer tails and fight your look. If this is a problem, keep things simple with plain studs. If you use clip-ons miss them out altogether. Accessorise the hair with ribbons and clips instead.

Side Sweeps: give you an asymmetric look by moving the hair from one side to the other. Likewise, if you part on one side and toss long hair over your head and clip or pin so that one ear is exposed. This looks very classy with longer hair over one shoulder and showing the nape and ear on the other side. The trick this time is to go for dangle and sparkle to balance that couture hair. The exposed ear will look gorgeous especially with a bare shoulder but don't make the earrings too long or big or you can destroy the asymmetry and make your face look longer.

In general, if you go for big or for detail in the hair accessories subdue the earrings. If the earrings are the centre of attention, subdue the hair accessories by going neutral. If you do want to treat yourself buy something with your birth stone. This can be a point of interest for a girly conversation or even a sharp-eyed man friend. Trust me though most men haven't a clue. Obviously, you can use your real birthday, but you might want to think about an alternative date that represents contacting or coming out with your inner girl. A trip out en-femme to browse the market and shops and pick up some jewellery or a choker can be great fun. All these little things help to express yourself fully. If you are not en-femme most people will think what you buy is a gift. No reason to feel self-conscious unless you forget and start holding them up to your ears.

Chokers (and what they mean)

We are not going to get into the wider world of jewellery selection. But one fashion accessory that is worth a mention is a choker. A strict definition of a choker is a close-fitting band or necklace worn around the neck as opposed to resting on the chest. Chokers are popular with transgendered women not just because they are associated with femininity but also because they hide or distract from the Adam's apple. A choker also provides a means of covering over any tidemark you leave after contouring your face. The downside is that chokers come with all sorts of symbology. So, let's take a little look at what you might be getting into:

<u>Ribbon chokers:</u> during the late 1800s chokers were worn by ballerinas and high-class women as ornamental statements. The thin ribbon can look very classy and highlight a thinner porcelain type neck. You might also like the look of ballet style hair (buns & braids) with cute close-fitting short cardigans and leggings or sweats over leotards. Personality wise a ribbon choker says you will be lively, energetic, open-minded, and easy to talk to. Be careful though, thin plain (red or black) ribbon perhaps with a little bow to one side were once confined to *fille de joie* (in modern parlance escorts, call girls, and so on.) These types can still mark you out as an easy girl or sexually promiscuous.

<u>Dog collars:</u> or more politely *colliers de chien* were popular in the early 1900s and incorporate all kinds of diamonds and pearls combined with lace and velvet. They were ornamental objects of the elite because apart from the stones they could be fitted perfectly to the neck and so became unique pieces. A wealthy dowager could wear one to display her worth or a debutante to show she was of marriageable age. Think Julia Roberts in *pretty woman*, dripping with stones when she goes to the opera, or a simple slim black velvet choker with a cute decoration at the centre (aka *Cinderella* in Disney's 1950s movie).

<u>Bondage collars:</u> the obvious example is the leather collar but there are many variations with buckles, studs, spikes, rings, or lockable silver

metal ones. Traditionally wearing a collar is highly significant in the BDSM scene and binds the submissive to the dominant. In recent years though it has become more mainstream as an accessory for naughty bedroom fun or for goths, punks and other edgy fashion looks. Check out the character, Abby Scuito, in the hit TV series *NCIS* for a variety of examples. Cat collars with little bells are also in this category which are bondage lite and can be a cute everyday look. Softer thinner collars are more feminine than the more edgy heavy ones, which hint at butch qualities. So, in a not so subtle way, you can show your persuasion as a top or bottom.

Sissy chokers: typically, these are wider styles that are very feminine and girly with oodles of lace and ribbons. But they can also be leather bondage style except in pink or barbie-like colours with hearts, rings, or sparkle. Simpler ribbon ones with lacy ruffs are often used with cosplay outfits like French Maids and sexy Bo peep. So, do not be surprised if you are being feminized or sissified and Mistress wants you to wear a choker with a pithy tag, motto, or motif.

Fashion chokers: are more mainstream and are just like a normal accessory. So, if you fancy the look but want to avoid the above references, this is what you need:

Silk: this is just like a plain piece of wider ribbon (half an inch to an inch). Its simplicity is the key and you can get away with them at work or as something a little different when socialising. Generally, they indicate a determined character but also someone that has a softer femme side.

Velvet: is like silk but has a little more class. Wider ones can cover a reasonable Adam's apple especially if you have an understated item of jewellery on the front. They are also soft and flexible enough to allow some movement. They sort of hint at wealth and finishing school. So, the image to project is one of sensuality and correctness. Good posture is essential to carry this look– shoulders back and upright torso, which will put your boobs a little bit out there (but don't arch your back).

Charms: in this style the main point of the choker is to support a charm or pendant type item. They are usually narrow, and the material can range from a leather strap to a thin metal hoop. A more bohemian or gypsy style with understated decorative pieces can look disarmingly cute. For example, unicorns, fairies, beads, or small feathers attached to a shoelace string.

Tattoos: use a tattoo sleeve designed for the neck. The material is always malleable so is easy to wear over your Adam's apple and varies from leather to plastic and metal weave. This allows for intricate 'inked' patterns of various thickness to adorn the neck. Thin simple ones are girly cute but thicker ones can give you a more edgy feel.

Lace: these are incredibly soft and feminine but differentiated from sissy chokers by using more subdued understated frills and neutral colours like black, white, cream and mauve. The emphasis is on delicacy and prettiness. They can vary from just a simple band of plain lace to velvet bands with lace ruffles. The former is dainty and the latter thicker covering like a ruff (or a scrunchy for your neck). The central area can be embellished further with dangles, jewellery, and ribbon which will give good coverage of the Adam's apple.

Statement pieces: these build on the above ideas with the band decorated in various ways using jewellery, patterns, beads, width and chunkiness (as in African or South American looks), very thick metal pieces, cut out chains or themes like gothic imagery. You can also go ultra-thin and delicate with just a hoop of silver or gold metal or thick cut with rings for pendants like an Ankh. Anything you can think of really to complement the rest of your look.

Obviously, the ability to carry this off depends on your neck. Longer necks can take thicker chokers but also look adorable with super thin ones. For shorter necks keep the width of the band to a third of your neck length or less. If you like the idea of masking the Adam's apple or your makeup but do not have a choker at hand think about using a scarf. Tie it in a neckerchief style with the knot to one side. This can look classy with plain silk and neutrals (think Audrey Hepburn) or more hippie or bohemian with tie-dyed materials.

Most mainstream on-line accessory shops will carry a range of chokers. If you want more specialist ones then you will need to look at adult stores, bondage shops, or crossdressing outlets. You are looking under £/$10 for a mainstream fashion style, £/$10-100 for bondage/sissy depending on the quality. A little plain leather style cat collar can be just as chic as a full metal bondage style, sissy ruff or something dripping with stones. The sky is the limit for full jewel/diamond ones. Depends on your look and personality. If you like this look there are lots to choose from and your only problem will be deciding what to buy. Browse away.

A choker fits snugly but should not squeeze the neck so include a bit extra for slack. You should be able to feel it is there (which is a nice girly reminder) but not be uncomfortable. Any faintness or difficulty in breathing take it off straight away. That sounds dramatic but if you are out and about and get hot or suddenly exert yourself your neck can swell. It is also why a mistress should not leave you alone if you are playing domination games. Bondage ones normally are adjustable but fashion ones maybe not. Oh, and don't think you can do this on the cheap either. Like from the pet store. A fully grown adult cat has a neck size of 10-12 inches and most dogs are similar. The human male neck has a circumference of 14-19 inches with the average about 15 inches. Most female chokers are between 14-16 inches so measure your neck beforehand and add a bit. Enough said.

Best Glasses for your face type

For many people it will be essential to wear corrective eyeglasses even when feminized. So, what can we learn about choosing the correct glasses to complement everything else? Well the first thing is that male and female glasses are different. Although there are unisex glasses around these are usually quite bland. And, of course, in the last few years men have started to become more fashion conscious so you can perhaps have more jazzy frames than previously. But, leaving all that aside, just like hair styles, glasses have their own gender. If you don't believe me try picking out different male and female sunglasses. For men we have the typical metal aviator style compared to pink, baby blue, or patterned frames for women. So, sweetie, you cannot just continue to wear your male glasses.

Male and female glasses differ in four main ways: frame size, lens shape, surrounding frame, and colour. Because men have different face structures to women there will always be a difference in the frame size. This is because the bridge of the nose is wider and the brow arch deeper. As a result, male frames often have different centre cushions and a straighter upper frame that runs along the brow ridge. Because the supraorbital eye structure is different between males and females, with female eyes a little bigger than male ones, you will find that men favour squarer or more rectangle lenses and lens holders whereas women like rounder lenses and softer frame shapes. Colour wise, men tend to go for darker neutral colours whereas women like lighter and more striking colours, two tone contrasts and patterns. A woman though is much more like to vary her choice of colour and frame so if she does go neutral, for work say, she is more likely to choose black, red, or dark blue frames. Men on the other hand tend to go brown, wood effect or metallic.

Here is a little guide based on your face shape to help choose your girl glasses:

Round Shaped Faces: are basically circles so we need to choose frames and lenses that are as wide as they are tall. This will make the face more oval and look slimmer. The lens frames need to be less round and/or have strong angles and not so big that they rest on the top of the cheeks. Vibrant prints, patterns, and colours, or embellishments that add contrast will also be good at taking away too much roundness.

Oval Shaped Faces: these again have lots of choices. For frame size the key is to choose one that runs slightly longer than the widest part of the face but not so big that it upsets the natural balance of the face. You can choose rectangular frames for a more professional look, cat-eye embellishments for a retro 1950/60s look, or a more artsy square or rounder frame. Since in this face type your cheekbones may be higher than other faces types you can also get away with all sorts of patterns and statement fashion bits.

Heart Shaped Faces have wide foreheads so as usual the glasses should help reduce this and try to make the chin look a little wider. Frames that are wider than your forehead will work, and you can distract with fancy endpoints which then lead the eye onto the contour of the face. A roundish lens will also help curve the face giving it a more oval look.

Square Shaped Faces: have those strong jawlines and straight features so we want to femme them up with curves and soft angles. You can make your face look less square by choosing frames that are wider than they are tall and using warm neutral colours like beige and cream. Anything that is not a dark male colour. Also avoid patterns that will add angles to your look. Lens wise use more rounder shapes to break up the angles of your face. Think about rimless glasses.

Oblong Shaped Faces: are longer than they are wide and might have proportionally higher cheekbones. The trick here is to go for lens frames that are higher than they are wide. Likewise use broad frames that have decoration at the temples and different colour on top of the rims. This may sound contradictory but what it will do is offset other long features like your nose or ears and make your face more proportional (remember the rule of thirds) and so appear less oblong. If your face is in proportion but just long use the frame width to create a more oval shape by pushing out the temple to cheek area.

Diamond Shaped Faces are narrow or pinched at the top and bottom with prominent wide cheeks. Thus, the eye line may look narrower than other face types. The trick here is to work with those cheekbones by using more angular frames. Use a wider overall frame to bring out the forehead area and use some patterns or colours. This will distract from your wide cheeks and focus attention on your eyes and eye makeup. Use more open lenses and avoid narrow lens frames which will just make your eyes look smaller.

The main point here is that if you want to have the widest choice of frames and go for those softer girl frames then you need to work on hair and face contouring to give you a more femme shape before you choose your glasses. Oh, and remember to choose colours that work with your eyes, skin tone and hair colour. We discussed all that in part 2. Note however that your choice for glasses needs to also complement your final choice for eyeshadow. If you order the wrong type of glasses, you may be stuck with a limited choices of shadow colours. That is why plain neutral frames often work better even though they might sound a little boring. Unless of course you buy multiply sets of glasses.

Finally, if a trip to the opticians to choose a set of girl frames is just too much, you can always order femme glasses online. Usually all you need is your prescription numbers for the lenses and then the world is your oyster. Choose the frames and design what your inner girl wants. Just like the virtual makeover apps there are many on-line platforms that allow you to try before your buy. So have fun. Ideally, femme up and then use that pic to choose your glasses. For an extra treat, when you pay on-line, send them to your femme self by just adding Ms or Miss, your girl name or initial to your own surname on the 'deliver to' address. Choosing your girl name is another whole topic in feminization but that will give you an extra buzz when they arrive. Assuming, of course, that there are no other family members or flat mates that will be curious. If that is the case hire a PO box for deliveries. If you have the will there is always a way.

Contacts and Doll eyes

If you just hate wearing glasses or want your girl persona to be glasses free you can use contact lenses. However, modern-day contacts can do more to feminize your features than just dropping the geek. You can give those irises and pupils some extra pep or choose colours that go better with your hair colour. Big pupils are also seen as more alluring, mostly because our pupils dilate when we are attracted to someone. Remember those renaissance beauties and the belladonna. The pupil is around 2-4mm in the light but can expand up to 8mm in the dark. That doesn't sound like a lot, but it is double normal size and very noticeable. Bigger irises can also be both stunning and disarming making you look adorable and cute. These are often called Doll eyes because they mimic the big fully lashed eyes on the dolls that girls play with when they are growing up.

Leaving drugs or medicines aside, there are various ways to make your pupils bigger. For example, picturing someone you find a turn-on, focusing on a distant object, or stressful situation. Butterflies in your tummy also work so try working your abdominal muscles. The more occupied your brain is the more your eyes will dilate. So, if you get involved with emotional processing too that will affect your pupil size. Lowering the lights, though, is probably the most reliable natural method because your eyes dilate in the dark to let in more light. If you ever wondered why gentleman's clubs and single bars tend to have subdued lighting, now you know. Red is often seen as a warm sexy or romantic colour and the staple of bordellos and such like, but it is an urban myth that the red light makes your eyes dilate more. In fact, your eyes do not dilate at all in red light. That is why they are used in submarine control rooms so you can switch to normal light when you go outside and back without affecting your eyes.

Anyways, contact lenses come in two varieties, cosmetic and circle lens. With a cosmetic contact lens, you can change your eye colour quite easily. Various transparencies let your own colours through and can add different tints, tones, or shades of your own eye colour for a little more contrast and pop. Opaque ones allow you to change your iris colour completely. Some people just use more intense versions of their own natural eye colour or you can go from ice blue to chocolate brown in a second and widen your choice of eye makeup. The inner edge of the iris area can also be coloured black for a bigger pupil which changes the contrast and context relationship with makeup colours. Ideal if you want to change things up or match an outfit.

Circle lenses are between 14-20mm in size which is much bigger than a normal contact and help create that doll eye look. Think Lady Gaga in the video for *Bad Romance*. The idea is that they extend the iris over the eye whites to give you bigger looking eyes. However, they also compromise the oxygen flow to your cornea. You will need to use eyedrops and only wear them for short periods. But if you want to look cutesy cute like anima or manga girls or barbie while you are en-femme and play or go clubbing these will do the job. There are a huge variety of colours and styles. If you are into cosplay then you can also get weird eyes, like all white, or all black, cat's eyes, or any colour you would care to mention. This way you can match your eye colour to any shade of hair and then match your eye shadow and outfits accordingly.

Putting it all together

We have seen all the techniques now, so for the last time let us put all this in perspective. In Part 1 we learned all about the underlying face shape and how everyone is on a spectrum between a stereotypical male or female face. We learned about face types and how people throughout the ages have tried to define beauty in the female form. All this gave us a yardstick to measure how feminine your face is and then some hints about how you can give any face a more feminine look. We also talked about all the tools and products needed to make that happen.

In Part 2 we developed a process to makeup up your face. We started by explaining how to cover those hard to hide male features and to prime the face for makeup proper. After that we learned how to contour the face to make it more typically female by cutting off angles to leave you closer to the classic oval shaped face which all women desire. We looked at how to use different skin-tones, highlighters, blush, and bronzers to give you face a more female profile by creating adorable cheeks and downplaying the brow bone and other bits. Next it was eyes and all you needed to know about eye makeup and colour contrast to get the look you want. After that we considered ways to make the mouth smaller, pouty, and fuller.

In Part 3 we added to all that by looking at hairpieces, wigs, and extensions exploring what they have to offer and a few do's and don'ts. We learned the vocabulary of hair and the various ways you can style and accessorise to give yourself a lovely feminine look. In framing your face, we learned how the shape of hair can work with your face type and what different cuts and styles may say about your femme persona. Finally, we looked at some extra add-ons that will help perfect your look including tips for the more mature girl, advice on choosing jewellery, glasses, and some quick styling tips that work in just about any circumstance.

Whatever your look, it is vitally important that you get in touch with your inner girl. We have said this many many times in these pages. If you feel congruent in yourself your girl time will be super rewarding. Listen to her and how she wants to be. You will be so emotionally satisfied when you get this right. And she will enjoy all the time you spend in front of the mirror, at the makeup table, or browsing for girl stuff. One way to work this is by going backwards through the book. Start with your femme personality and then choose the right hair style and length, then the makeup eye colours and lippy to match, and then decide how much contouring you are going to need. If you want a more natural look then you will need less. If you want to go for a complete makeover, you will need to do more. Once you have your look begin to practice putting on your face.

At the start of the book we talked about being passable and set that as an objective for occasional girls. If all you want is to do is enjoy girl time in your own home and dress while you do household jobs, watch TV, do hobbies, or pamper yourself that is one thing. You can get by with less make up effort because the key is to feel happy inside. If you do want to go out, shopping say, or for a coffee, to meet other 'girls', or just enjoy a cinema trip or a walk in the park you will need to do more. In these cases, you will need to matchup your whole ensemble, develop some of the female gestures and body language we talked about, and generally just deport yourself in a female way. Your goal here should be twofold. First is to avoid any obvious 'tells' so you can melt into the crowd and go about enjoying girl time without any hassle or hesitant looks. And second is to be so natural that guys hold the door open for you and when you buy stuff or ask about things people call you Miss, Ms, or Ma'am. When that happens, you will feel a flip of excitement inside and smile on your lips.

And Finally

Well that is it, darlings! Another set of tools in your quest to become the best girl you can. I do hope you have found all the above useful. If you have a better understanding of the female face and the techniques you can use, that is a win. Take what you need and leave the rest. Hair and makeup are vast topics but still only covers one of the four pillars of feminization. If you have found this book useful and informative then have a look at the sister volumes listed at the back where you can find out all about feminizing your body and your voice.

We spent a lot of time on vocabulary and techniques so now you should be fully equipped to browse online or read magazines and understand the tips and methods used for the looks you might like. And, more importantly, be able to buy the right things for the femme you. The resources section lists a few websites that will help with virtual makeovers, finding the right hair pieces, and getting the right looks. Remember though that your inner girl has her own personality. Enjoy sitting in front of the makeup mirror and experimenting.

If you find that you just love the world of makeup and hair and that you are good at it, or you are sought after by your other girlfriends, consider taking a beauty or a hair styling course. Not only is this a lovely feminine pastime but you can get certificates that will allow you to charge for your time and effort or do makeovers. It is a great way to socialise. Just a thought.

Anyways, whatever you do, good luck. And, always remember the words of that paragon of fashion and style – Coco Chanel:

A girl should be two things classy and fabulous.

Ciao for now.

Resources

Some places to keep your feminization alive and to find obscure things. A listing here does not imply endorsement– you surf and shop on-line at your own risk. Not all places are crossdressing aware. Please be polite and discreet when contacting or ordering. All URLs last checked 10/10/20. You can also check YouTube for many many specific makeup tutorials including male-to-female ones. There are also lots of makeup products and accessories on amazon, ebay, and similar places for low prices.

Big name virtual try ons
https://www.lorealprofessionnel.co.uk/hair-looks/style-my-hair
https://www.chanel.com/en_GB/fragrance-beauty/makeup/c/chanel-try-on.html
https://www.loreal-paris.co.uk/virtual-try-on
https://www.maybelline.com/virtual-try-on-makeup-tools
https://www.bobbibrown.co.uk/virtual-try-on

hairstyle and virtual makeovers
https://www.thehairstyler.com/
https://stylecaster.com/virtual-makeover/
https://www.easyhairstyler.com/
https://www.instyle.com/makeover/makeover-tool

Professional concealers, correctors, and more
https://camerareadycosmetics.com/
https://makeupprostore.co.uk/
https://thedragqueencloset.com/

Wigs
https://www.wigstoreuk.co.uk/
https://www.celebwigs.com/
https://procrossdresser.com/
https://hairsleisure.com/

Contacts & Doll eyes
https://www.pinkyparadise.com/
https://www.uniqso.com/

Vintage Makeup & Looks
https://vintagedancer.com/
https://vintagemakeupguide.com/
https://hair-and-makeup-artist.com/

Miscellaneous face reading and style

https://www.kendrapowell.com/blog/the-5-golden-metrics-for-your-true-eye-shape
http://lipsology.com/
https://www.yourchineseastrology.com/

More Feminization Books by Martine

How To Feminize Your Body, 2020, pp176

ISBN-13:979-8614947729, ASIN:B084WV3DYQ

The topic is male-to-female transformation. Some people call it makeover, that works too. The text is written predominantly from the view that you are new to crossdressing and feminization but want to develop a female persona of some kind be it permanent or just for a temporary indulgence. If you are an old hand then you may also find a few helpful tips or insights that will further enhance your look, style, or dressing technique. An assumption is that you were not socialised as a girl. As a result, we need to revisit and spend time on all the little things females seem to find so natural and take for granted. Getting in touch with your femininity is a mixture. An ensemble if you will of lots of things. When you see an ultra-feminine woman, the way she acts and dresses, the way she walks and talks, and oozes sensuality you know there is something more going on than just putting on a dress.

How To Feminize Your Voice, 2019, pp126

ISBN13:9781794084179, ASIN: B07M85MTPY

You have gone to the trouble of getting your figure all curvy. Dressed right for your body type. Done your hair and makeup. You look great – what next? Do you have a naturally sexy husky voice or is it more night club bouncer? Imagine what it would be like to sound naturally more femme? Voice feminization is a growing phenomenon within the crossdressing and transgender community. This no-nonsense book provides all the tricks, tips, and advice you will need to create a passable feminine voice. No surgery required. Learn the four big secrets that will make the most difference to your voice: tone, resonance, rhythm, and word choice. Use these techniques and you will create a female voice that not only sounds femme but also matches your personality. Each chapter makes it easy to learn by giving you a little theory, practice exercises, as well as common mistakes to avoid. Whether you want a temporary or permanent adjustment or are simply curious to find out how females speak differently to men you will be sure to find something of interest inside.

Made in the USA
Columbia, SC
29 June 2025